TIME TO RELAX

SELF-CARE

ACTIVITY BOOK

BY: BRIDGETT MCGILL

ALL RIGHTS RESERVED. NO PARTS OF THIS BOOK MAY BE REPRODUCED OR TRASNMITTED IN ANY FORM OR BY ANY MEANS, ELECTRONIC OR MECHANICAL, INCLUDING PHOTOCOPYING, RECORDING OR BY ANY INFORMATION STORAGE OR RETRIEVAL SYSTEMS, WITHOUT PERMISSION IN WRITING FROM THE COPYRIGHT OWNER.

COPYRIGHT @ NOVEMBER 2024 BY BRIDGETT MCGILL / THE QUEEN WITHIN

ISBN: 978-1-7367830-9-2

OTHER WORKS BY THIS AUTHOR:

- *HOW DOES YOUR GARDEN GROW? CULTIVATING A LIFE OF ABUNDANCE*

- *HOW DOES YOUR GARDEN GROW? CULTIVATING A LIFE OF ABUNDANCE: THE INTERACTIVE JOURNAL*

- *BIRTHING PURPOSE: 21- DAY DEVOTIONAL JOURNAL*

- *REDEMPTION: SINS OF THE WINDY CITY SERIES*

- *CONCRETE BAYOU*

- *EMERGING QUEENS SELF-CARE JOURNAL FOR GIRLS*

COLLABORATIONS INCLUDE:

— *The Oil*
— *21- Day Devotional Journal*
— *My Self-Care Journal*
— *My Affirmations Journal*

DEDICATION

This book is dedicated to all my Sister-Queens and their individual, unique, self-care journeys.

To the Queen who has yet to understand the value in making herself a priority; say hello to self-care. You may not be there yet, but as you continue to move through this book you will see WHY you are so important. You will begin to pour into and validate yourself without any approval needed.

To the Queen who has just begun practicing self-care; welcome. Now that you have stepped onto your new path, the elevated woman who is waiting on the other side beckons you to keep moving forward and not look back. Access has been granted.

To the Queen who makes caring for herself a lifestyle; we applaud you and look to you to for guidance. Share with us how to go within and do real shadow work; to create a new life for ourselves. We see you glowing, and we want the tea.

Wherever you are in your self-care journey, give yourself a round of applause and be proud of you.

Queen Bea

This book belongs to:

_____

Self Care o'clock ♡

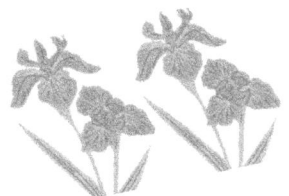

DAY ONE

EMOTIONAL INTELLIGENCE

"The capacity to be aware of, control and express one's emotions, to handle interpersonal relationships judiciously and empathetically."

REFLECTION: Our emotional intelligence is a part of who we are. Emotional intelligence shapes our personalities and thought processes. As we mature, learn and grow, our emotional intelligence should be continually increasing. How does your emotional intelligence show up in your life?

Self-Care Tip

Let's practice deep breathing. Take a deep breath, count to one, and exhale. Take the second deep breath, and exhale to the count of two. Take a third breath, exhale to the count of three, until your lungs are empty. For the fourth breath, inhale deeply, and exhale to the count of four until your lungs are completely empty. Take inventory of your body and see how you feel after each round of breaths. You can try this a couple of times a day, a few times a week. Deep breathing is one method that can be used to reset your body, slow your heart rate, clear your mind and regulate your emotions.

JOURNAL

_____

_____

_____

_____

_____

_____

Emotional Intelligence Day 1

Can you find the words hidden in the puzzle?

```
U N D E R S T A N D W D
P A R D E N T C S T U P
K S E R X O I U H A R I
N R E A S O N M C N I C
O P A S S I O N A T E N
W R S I P T T N C M K I
L S I Y T I I U M M O C
E A L E N T S R P R S F
D X P E R T I S R S U I
G P R O U S E D F E N E
E C O M P E T E N C D R
P E R S P I C A C I T Y
```

UNDERSTAND   FIERY   REASON   PERSPICACITY

KNOWLEDGE   ROUSED   ARDENT

ACUMEN   STIRRED PASSIONATE

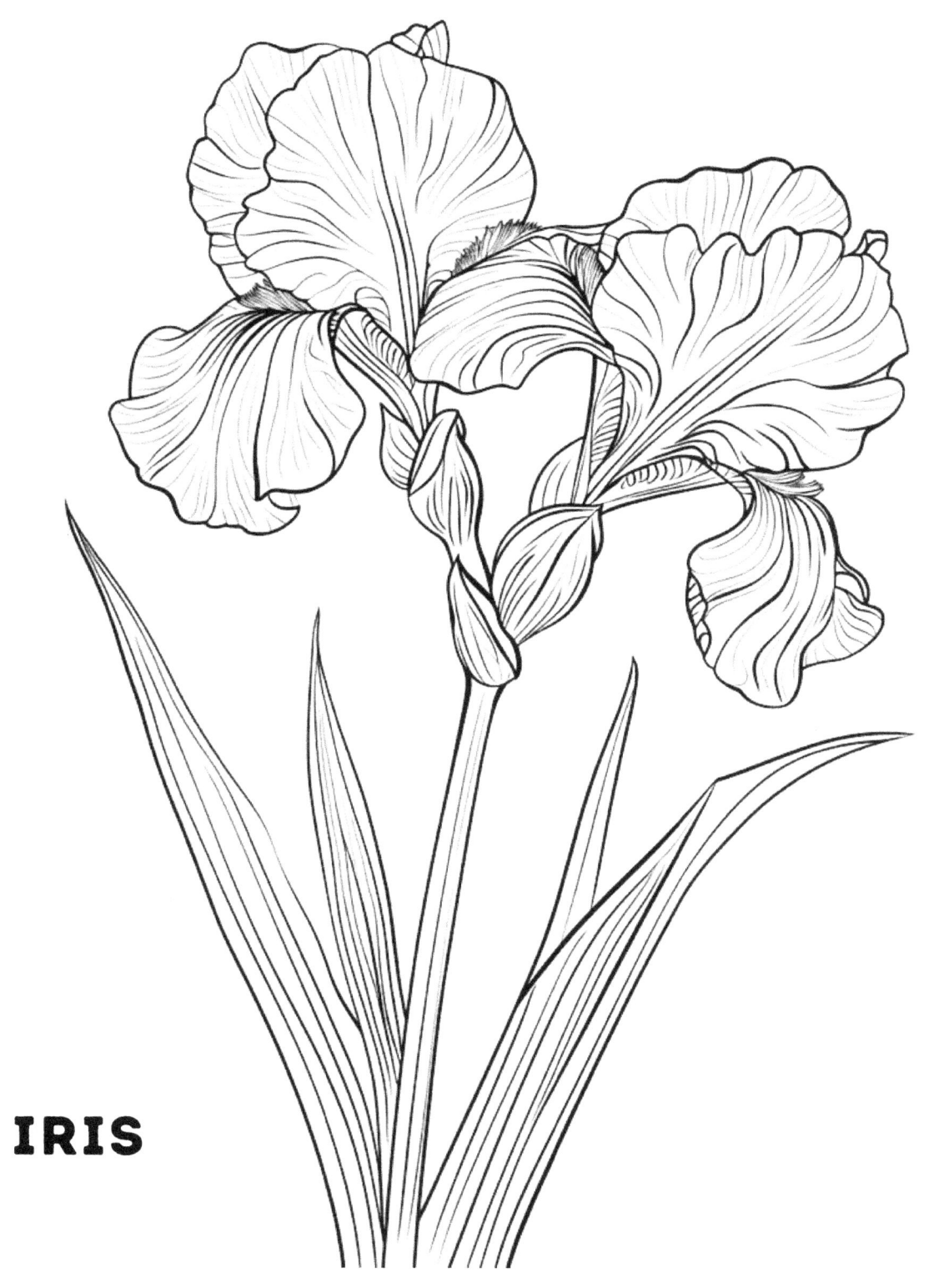

DAY TWO

SELF-AWARENESS

"The conscious knowledge of one's own character, feelings, motives, and desires."

REFLECTION: How aware are you of you? What makes you happy? Do you need to forgive yourself? Do you need to forgive anyone else? What is your level of pettiness? What are your triggers? Identify the areas in which you have grown and celebrate yourself.

 Self-Care Tip
Hug a tree today. Science says that hugging a tree can lower stress levels, reduce cortisol, decrease anxiety and lower your heart rate and blood pressure. Try it and write about your tree hugging experience.

JOURNAL

_____

_____

_____

_____

_____

_____

_____

_____

Awareness Day 2

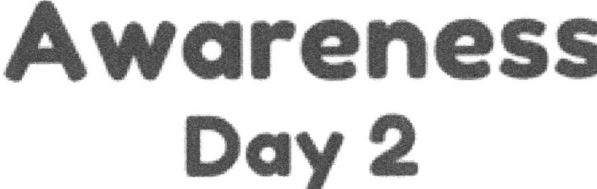

Can you find the words hidden in the puzzle?

```
R E C O G N I T I O N P
F S I G H T I C S T U E
A S E R X O I S H A R R
M E A A C I V I C N I C
I L T S S H A R E D C E
L R S P P N T T C M K P
I A P P R E C I A T E T
A A L E N T H G I S N I
R E A L I Z A T I O N O
T P R O W E S S F T N N
E G D E L W O N K C E N
R N D N A T S R E D N U
```

RECOGNITION   **PERCEPTION**   **FAMILIAR**   **UNDERSTAND**

REALIZATION   **GRASP**   **KNOWLEDGE**

SIGHT   **APPRECIATE**   **INSIGHT**

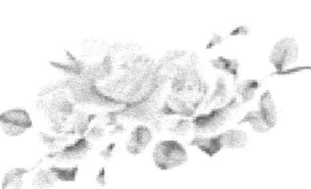

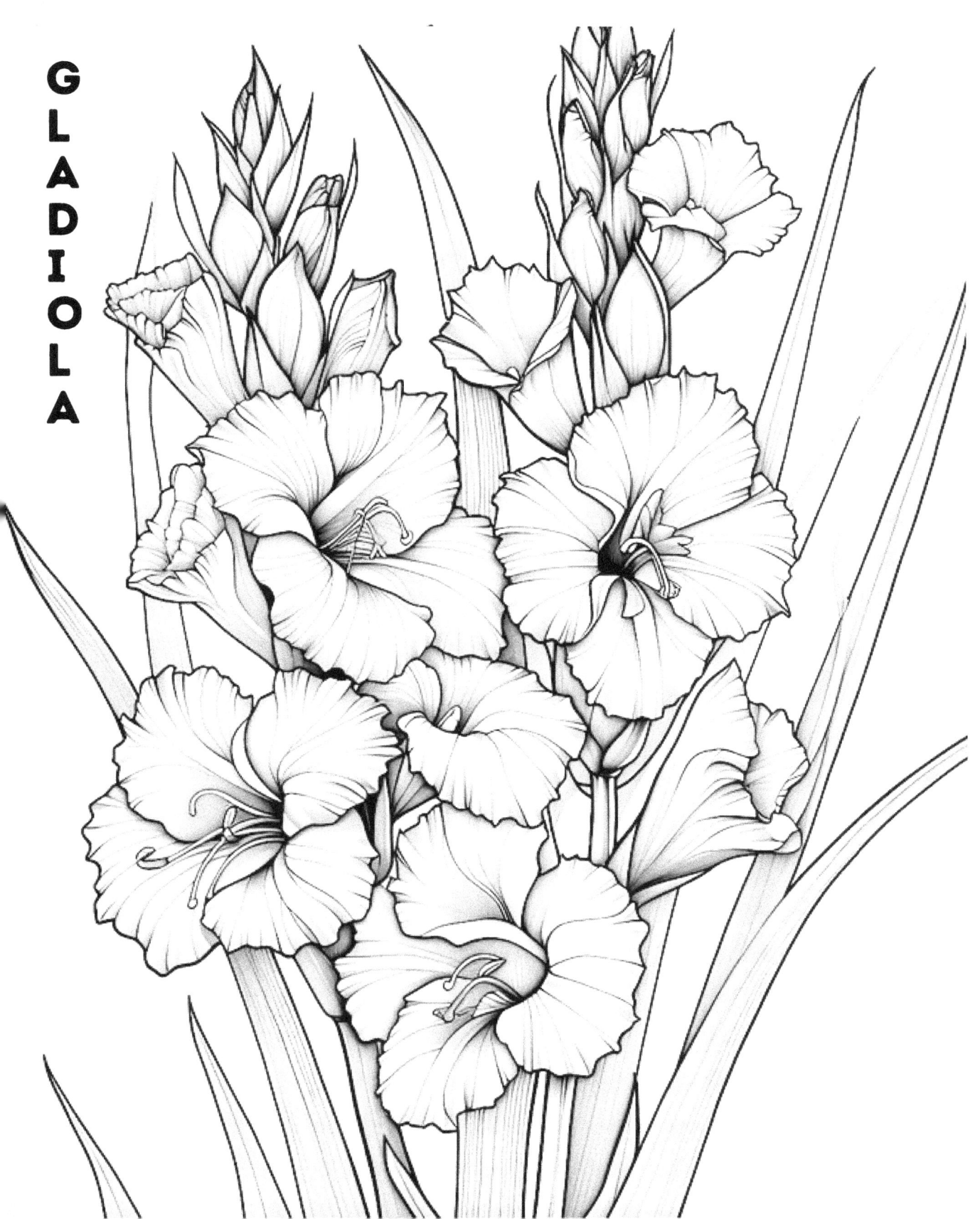

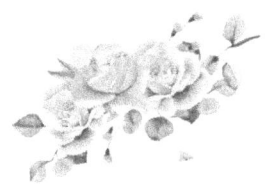

DAY THREE
SOCIAL SKILLS

"Ways of interacting with others that make it easier to succeed socially."

REFLECTION: Social skills are very important especially today. With the advancements in technology and travel, we have to be intentional with our words and actions to avoid unnecessary negativity. How do you interact in social situations with strangers? How do you behave when you are with your friends and family?

Self-Care Tip
It's a great day for a detox bath;

RECIPE:
1 cup baking soda, 1 cup peroxide, 1 cup Epsom salt

Mix the ingredients into a tub of hot water.

Soak for at least 20 minutes while speaking your favorite affirmations or prayers out loud.

Alternatively, you could simply relax and allow your body to detox.

Examples of Affirmations:
~Everything is working as it should, I am safe.

~ I love myself, I love my mind, I love my body and I am Worthy of respect.

~ I am a positive, happy person and my life is getting better every day.

JOURNAL: _____

_____

_____

_____

_____

_____

_____

_____

_____

_____

_____

_____

Social Skills Day 3

Can you find the words hidden in the puzzle?

```
C O M M U N A L B O W D
P A R T B L I C S T U P
U S E R X O I S H A R I
B E A N C I V I C N I C
L L T A S H A R E D C N
I R S I P N T T C M K I
C S I Y T I N U M M O C
T A L E N T S E P R S A
E X P E R T I S E S U N
T P R O W E S S F T N S
E C O M P E T E N C E N
R N I A B I L I T I E S
```

COMMUNAL   SHARED   TALENTS   PROWESS

PUBLIC   COMMUNITY EXPERTISE

CIVIC   ABILITIES COMPETENCE

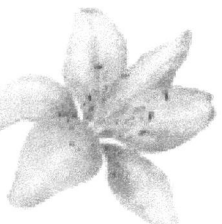

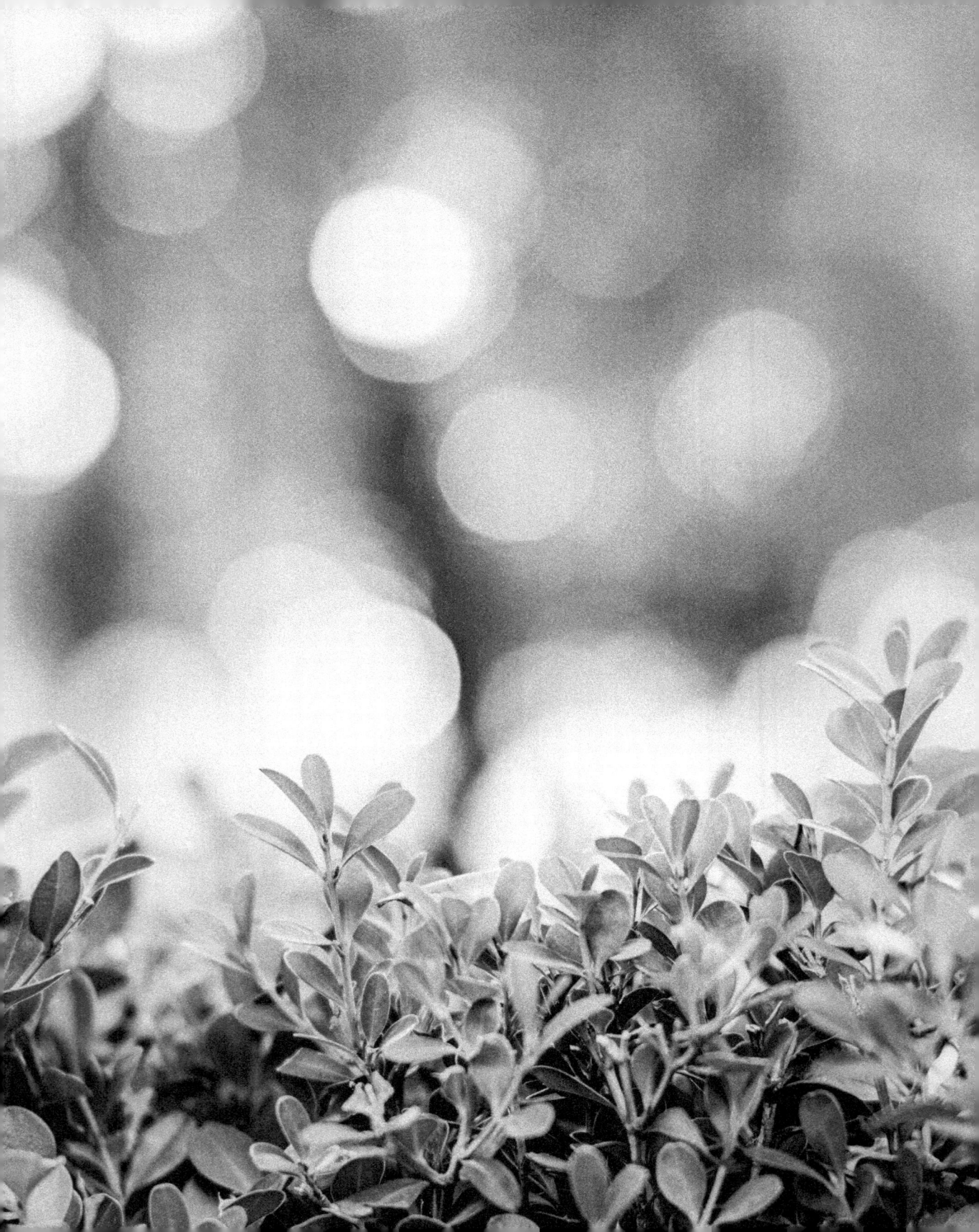

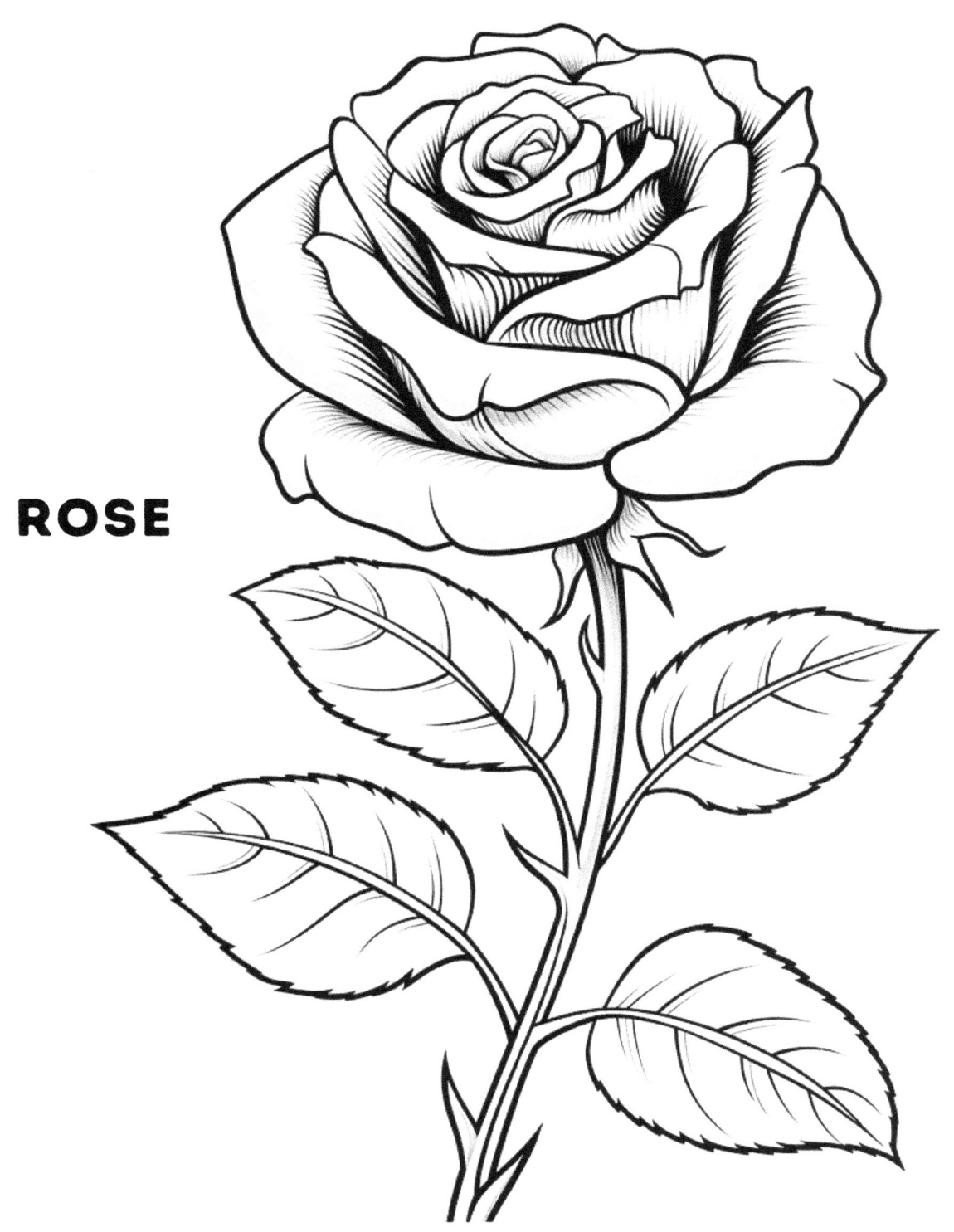

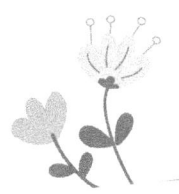

DAY FOUR
EMPATHY

"The ability to understand and share the feelings of another."

REFLECTION: Could you show more empathy to other people or yourself? Do you need more empathy from someone in your life? How would empathy improve your relationships?

 Self-Care Tip
Create your own anointing oil and anoint your home.

RECIPE:
1-part carrier oil (ex: olive oil, avocado oil, grape seed oil, coconut oil)

2-part essential oil (ex: Frankincense, peppermint oil, lavender oil or oil of your choice)

Anoint your doorways, windows, doorknobs while praying for protection, peace and covering over your home.

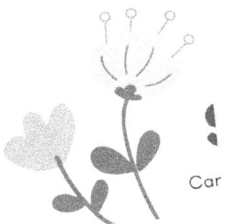

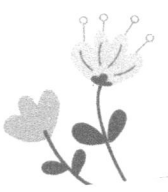

JOURNAL: _____

Empathy Day 4

Can you find the words hidden in the puzzle?

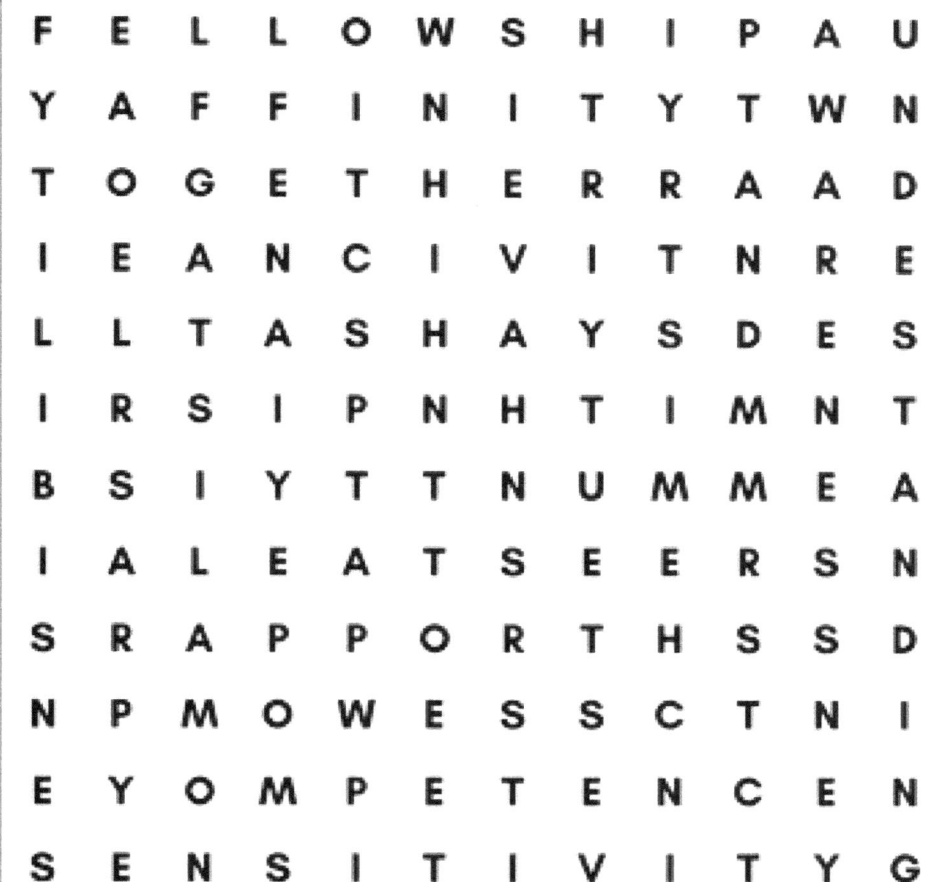

```
F E L L O W S H I P A U
Y A F F I N I T Y T W N
T O G E T H E R R A A D
I E A N C I V I T N R E
L L T A S H A Y S D E S
I R S I P N H T I M N T
B S I Y T T N U M M E A
I A L E A T S E E R S N
S R A P P O R T H S S D
N P M O W E S S C T N I
E Y O M P E T E N C E N
S E N S I T I V I T Y G
```

AFFINITY   UNDERSTANDING   AWARENESS   CHEMISTRY

RAPPORT   SENSITIVITY   FELLOWSHIP

SYMPATHY   SENSIBILITY   TOGETHER

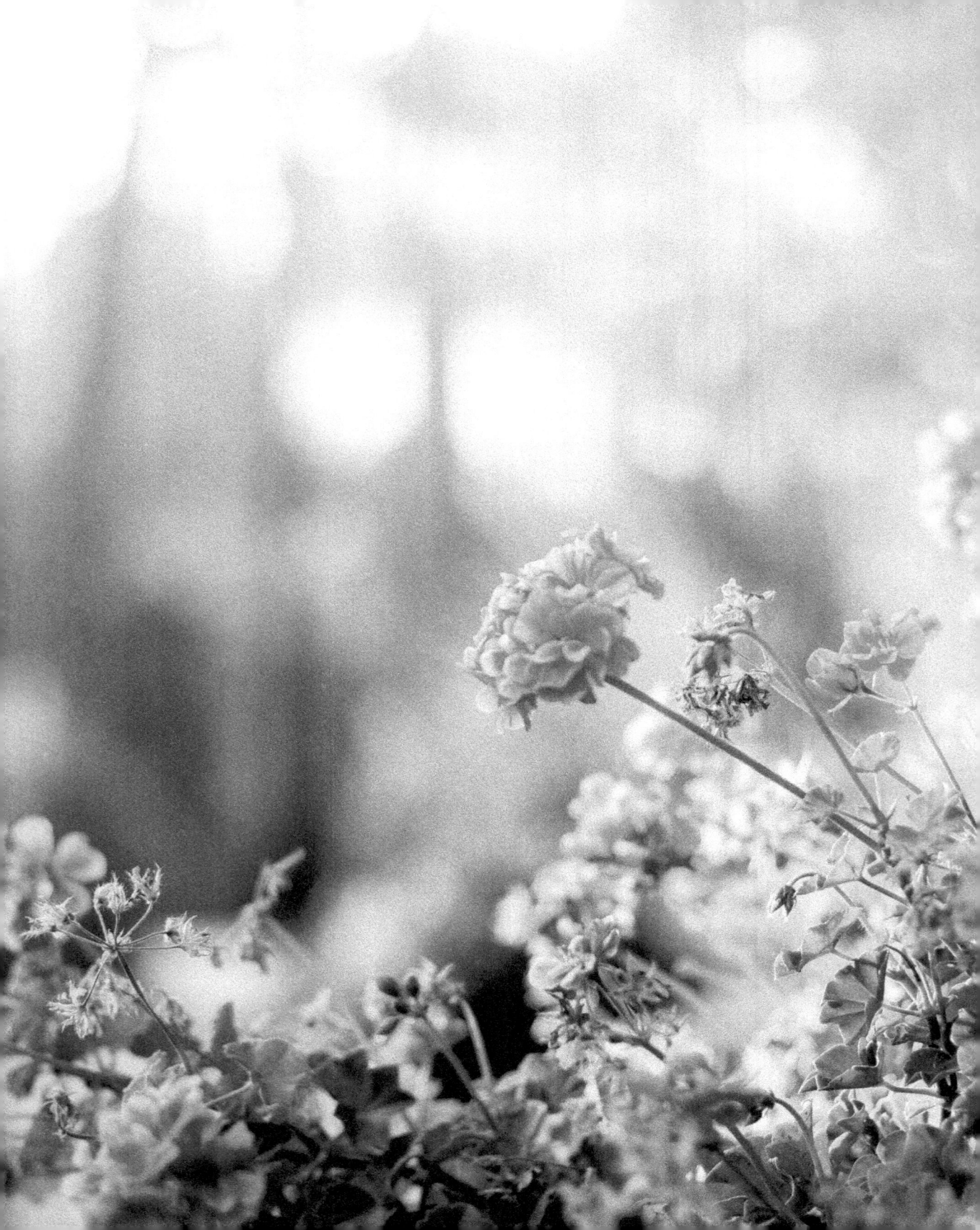

LILLY

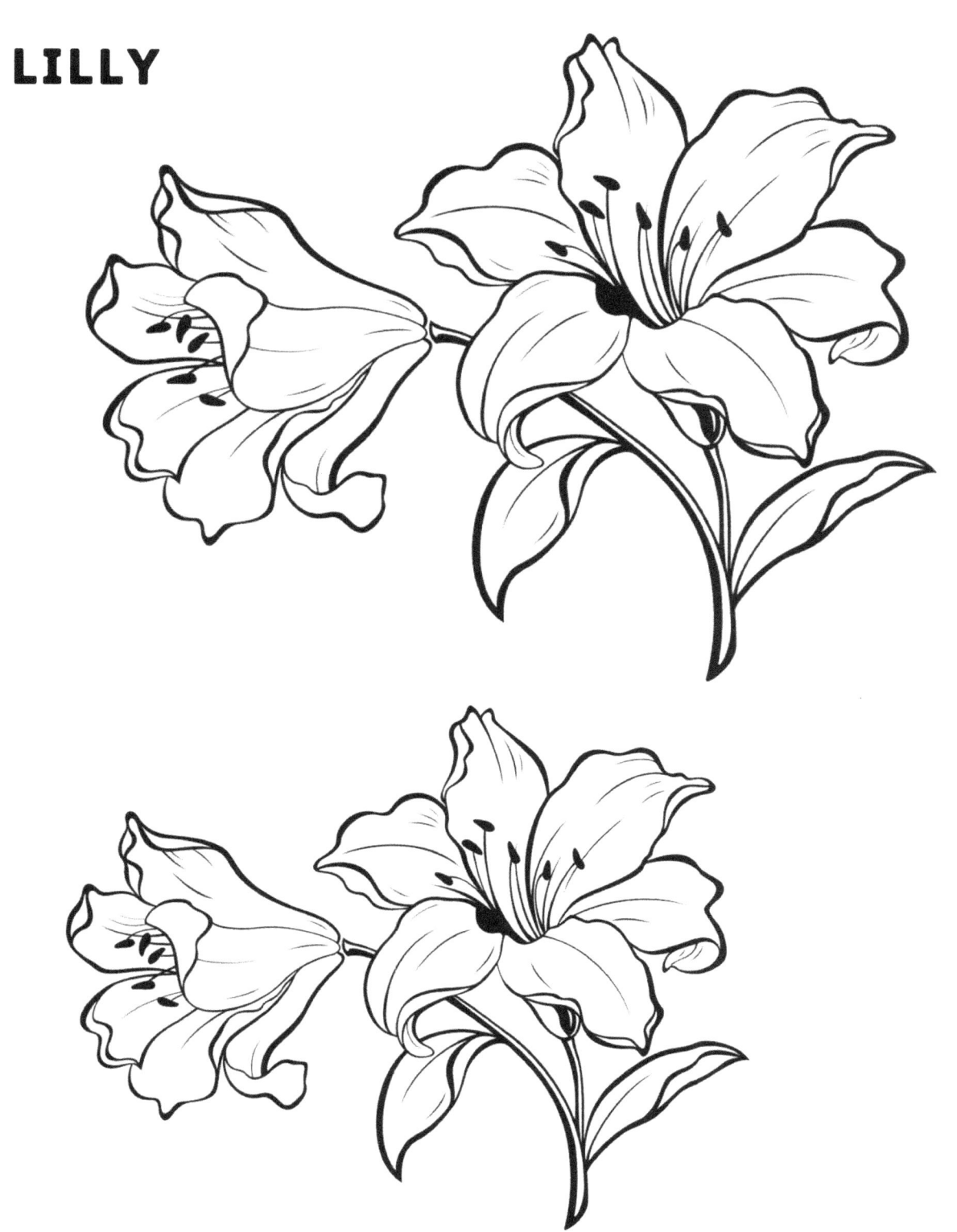

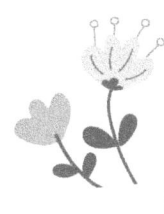

DAY FIVE

INTERNAL or INTRINSIC MOTIVATION

"Motivation that is defined as the intention to engage in a behavior because of the inherent satisfaction of the activity rather than the desire for a reward or specific outcome."

REFLECTION: What is your purpose? Who are you when you are alone and no one is looking at you? Do you consider yourself a good person?

Self-Care Tip Forward Fold Stretch.
Stand with feet slightly apart. Inhale lifting both arms above your head, exhale once palms are facing each other. Inhale a deep breath and then exhale as you slowly bend forward, bringing hands to floor; or as close to the floor as you can. Take a few deep breaths in the folded position. Next, take a deep breath and slowly exhale as you come up to a standing position with hands above your head and bring arms slowly down to your sides. Write down how you felt after this amazing spine stretch.

JOURNAL

_____

_____

_____

_____

_____

_____

_____

Motivation Day 5

Can you find the words hidden in the puzzle?

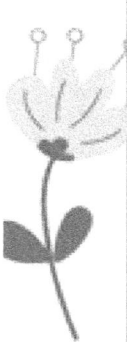

```
I N C E N T I V E S W D
I C A U S E M I S P U R
I N S P I R A T I O N I
N P U R N C M T S S I C
C L M I M P U L S E C N
E I S L M O T I V E K I
N U S I T M U L U S O C
I N D U C E M E N T S A
I I A I I T C P S E U N
V N T S O N R E A S O N
E I N C I T E M E N T N
S T I M U L U S A B Y E
```

INCENTIVE   SPUR   INCITEMENT   CAUSE

INSPIRATION   STIMULUS   INDUCEMENT

IMPULSE   MOTIVE   REASON

CHRYSANTHEMUM

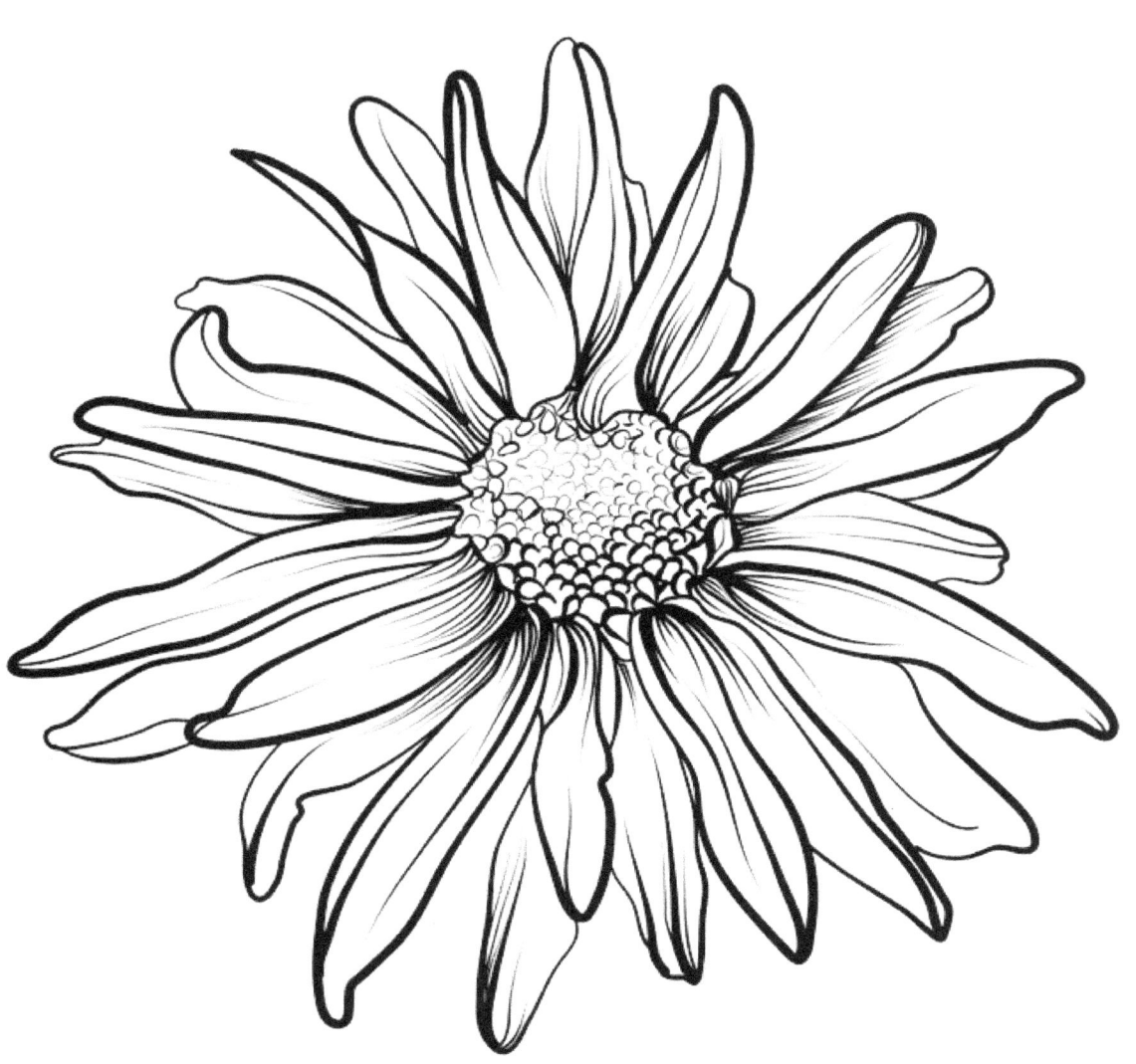

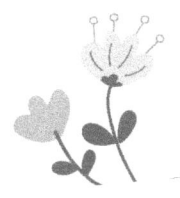

DAY SIX

SELF – REGULATION

"The ability to control one's behavior, and manage your thoughts and emotions. It involves being aware of your goals and progress and adjusting your actions accordingly."

REFLECTION: Keep your eyes on your prize. Be intentional about the conversations, environments and activities you allow yourself to participate in. Distractions disrupt our regulation and delay our destinies.

 Self-Care Tip
Cleansing and confession. Do you wash your face in the mirror? Today you're going to wash your face and then look at yourself, eye to eye and confess your sins, your shadows, your mistakes. It's just you, the mirror and your soul. After confession, wash your face again and forgive yourself and say it out loud. "I forgive myself for it all." Now walk out of the bathroom with less baggage holding you down and all you confessed down the drain.

JOURNAL

_____
_____
_____
_____
_____
_____

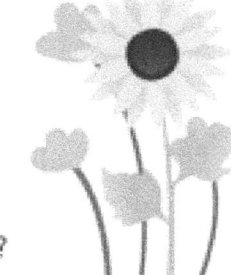

Regulation Day 6

Can you find the words hidden in the puzzle?

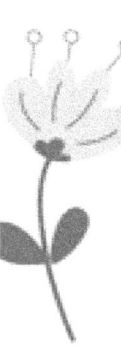

I	S	T	E	W	A	R	D	S	H	I	P
S	U	P	E	R	V	I	S	I	O	N	P
G	S	D	I	R	E	C	T	I	O	N	I
O	C	O	R	R	E	C	T	I	O	N	C
V	O	M	U	S	P	U	L	U	U	C	O
E	N	S	L	M	O	T	I	V	E	K	N
R	T	S	I	T	M	U	L	U	S	O	D
N	R	D	U	C	E	M	E	N	T	S	U
A	O	A	I	C	T	C	P	S	E	U	C
N	L	M	A	N	A	G	E	M	E	N	T
C	I	N	G	U	I	D	A	N	C	E	N
E	T	I	M	U	L	U	E	A	B	Y	E

STEWARDSHIP **CARE** **DIRECTION** **CORRECTION**

SUPERVISION **CONDUCT** **MANAGEMENT**

CONTROL **GUIDANCE** **GOVERNANCE**

SUNFLOWER

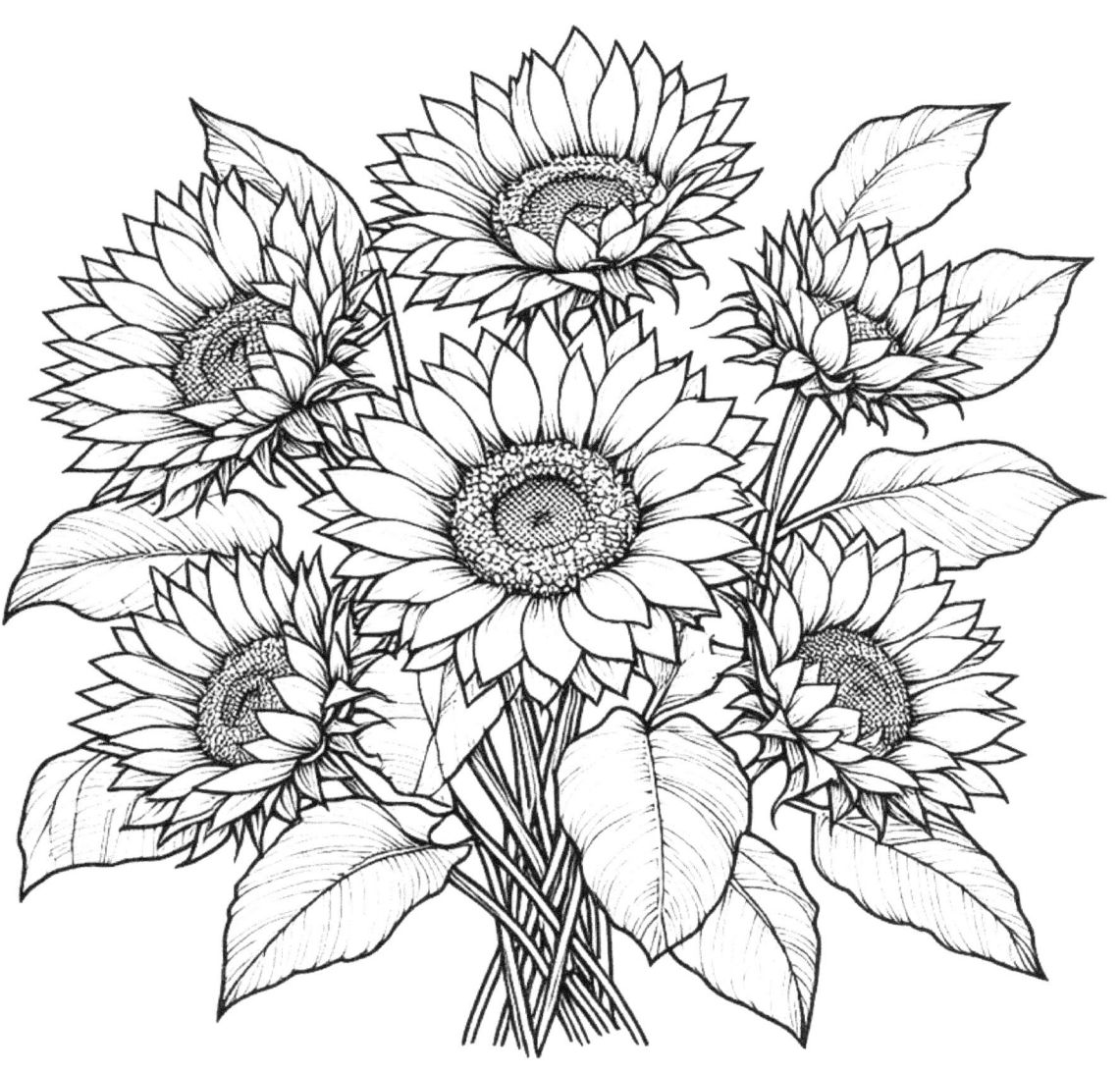

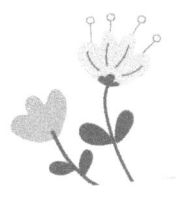

DAY SEVEN

PRIORITY

"The fact or condition of being regarded or treated as more important."

REFLECTION: There's no one more important in your life than you. If you are not well and whole, everyone who depends on you will not be either. For example: When you are on an airplane. Before the plane ascends into the air you are instructed by the stewardess,

"If you are with a small child or someone that may need assistance, put on your mask FIRST and then help them with their mask."

You have to be okay in order to help someone else. Have you ever heard the phrase,
"You can't pour from an empty cup."

Self-Care Tip
Set your clock for a Mid-night prayer. Usually this is a quiet, private time. You may need to go and find a place where you can sit alone for a few moments and communicate with your Higher Power. If you need to get out of bed, get up. Go sit on the couch or in the bathroom. Keep the light off if you can and use this time to pour your heart out to The Most High.

JOURNAL

_____

_____

_____

_____

_____

Priority
Day 7

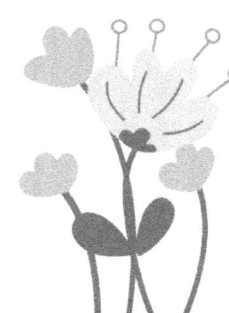

Can you find the words hidden in the puzzle?

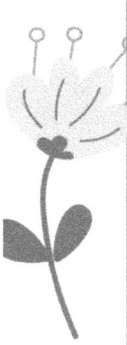

```
P R E E M I N E N C E P
R U E C N E D E C E R P
E S D I R E A N C E N I
F C U R G E N Y I O N C
E C N A C I F I N G I S
R N S L M G T I V E K N
E T S I R M U L U S O D
N R D U C E M E N T S O
C W E I G H T P K E U R
E I M P O R T A N C E D
C I N G U I R A N K A E
E T S E N I O R I T Y R
```

PRECEDENCE	URGENCY	PREEMINENCE	ORDER
IMPORTANCE	WEIGHT	PREFERENCE	
SIGNIFICANCE	RANK	SENIORITY	

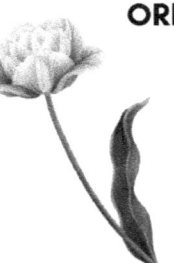

PEONY

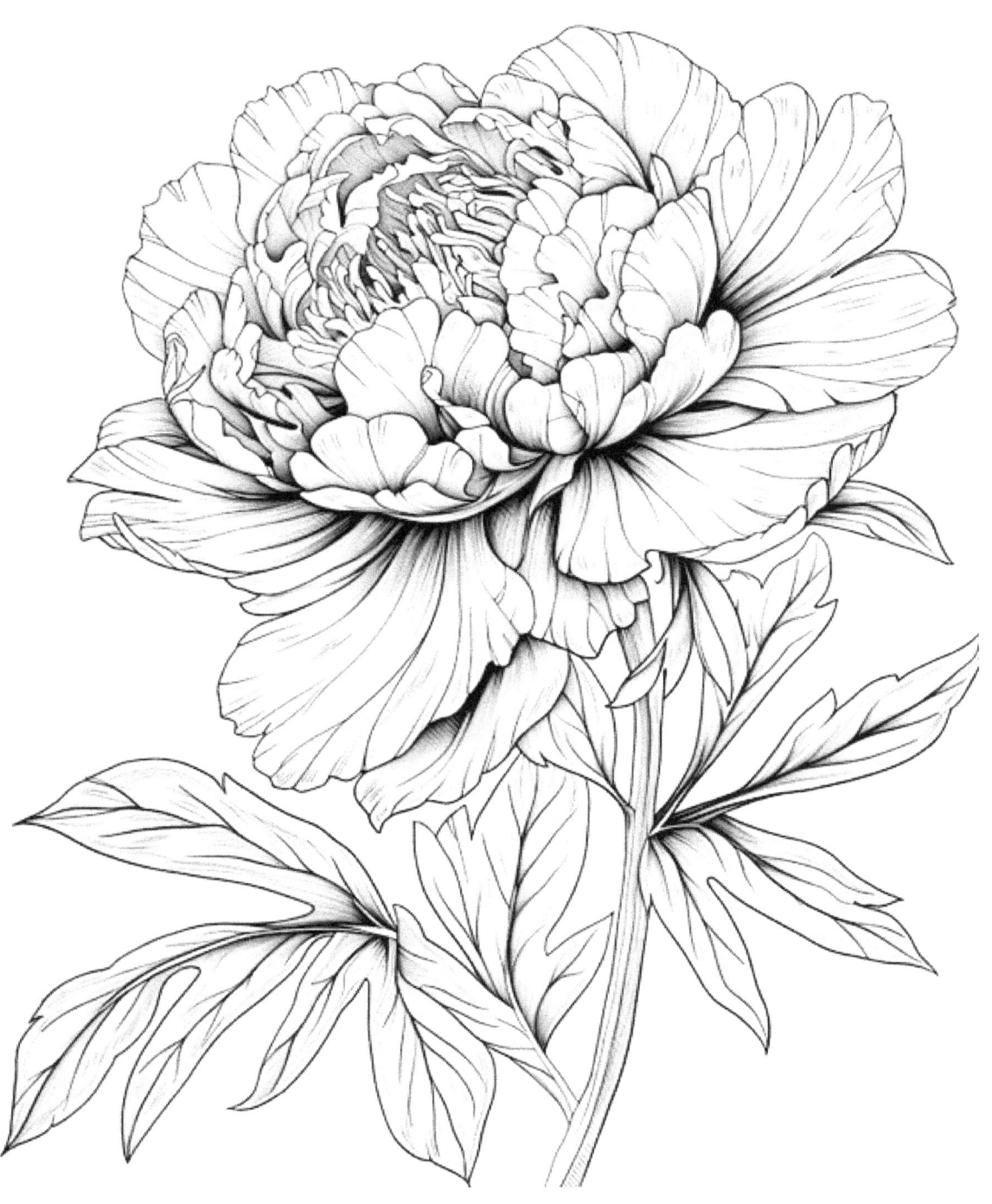

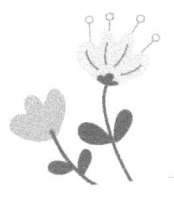

DAY EIGHT

PRESS

"To move or cause to move into a position of contact with something by exerting continuous physical force."

REFLECTION: The amount of oil in your life, depends on your level of press. To smooth out the rough parts of your life, you must apply pressure to the area. Push that negativity away from you, press through the heartache and come out on the other side. Press your life into the shape you dream of. Are you taking responsibility for your life and pressing with all your effort?

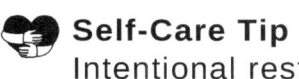
Self-Care Tip
Intentional rest

Make room in your day to take a nap. Even if you don't go to sleep. Get comfortable in your bed, take some deep breaths and allow your body to fully relax.

JOURNAL

_____
_____
_____
_____
_____
_____
_____

Press
Day 8

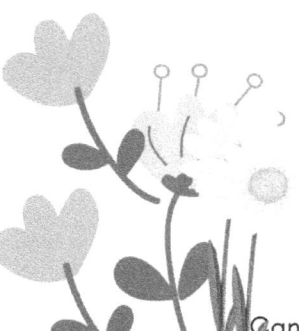
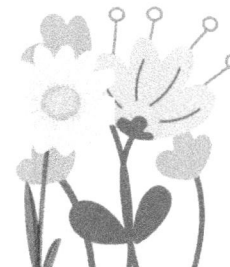

Can you find the words hidden in the puzzle?

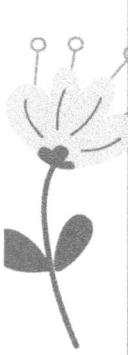

```
P R E E M I N E N C E P
R P M C B E A R D O W N
E I D O P U S H C E N I
F G U R V E H Y I O N C
E N N A C E O I N G I S
W I S L M G L I V E K N
E O S I R M D L U S O D
I N S Q U E E Z E T S O
G W E I G H T P K E U R
H C O M P R E S S C E D
O I S H A P E A N K A E
N T L E V E L R I T Y R
```

BEARDOWN	**HOLD**	**SQUEEZE**	**SHAPE**
PUSH	**MOVE**	**LEVEL**	
COMPRESS	**PIGNION**	**WEIGHON**	

DAISY

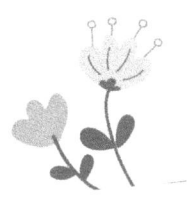

DAY NINE
INNATE

"Inborn; natural."

REFLECTION: You already have everything you need to do what you need to do. The Bible promises that you have the power to succeed. Notice 2 Peter 1:3 "His divine power has given us everything we need for a godly life through our knowledge of him who called us by his own glory and goodness."

 Self-Care Tip
Set aside some time today, preferably early in the morning and read a chapter from the bible or a book that adds to your personal toolbox. Journal about what you are reading and why. How will this reading material move you closer to your goals?

JOURNAL

_____

_____

_____

_____

_____

_____

Innate
Day 9

Can you find the words hidden in the puzzle?

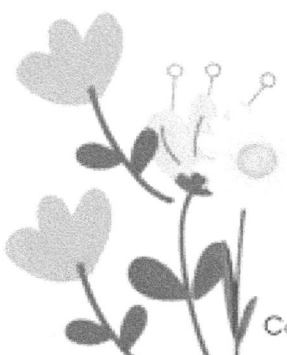
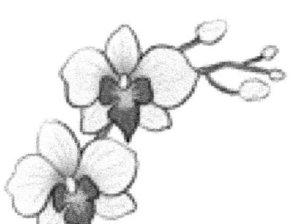

P	R	E	E	M	I	N	B	O	R	N	P
I	P	M	C	B	H	A	R	D	O	W	N
N	A	T	I	V	E	S	H	C	E	N	I
B	U	I	L	T	I	N	Y	I	O	N	C
R	N	N	A	C	E	O	I	N	G	I	I
E	I	S	L	M	N	A	T	U	R	A	N
D	O	S	I	R	T	D	L	U	S	O	H
I	N	T	E	G	R	A	L	E	T	S	E
G	W	E	I	G	H	T	P	K	E	U	R
H	E	R	E	D	I	T	A	R	Y	E	E
O	I	S	H	A	P	E	A	S	Y	A	N
N	T	C	N	I	T	S	N	I	T	Y	T

INHERENT   INTEGRAL   INBRED   INSTINCT
NATURAL   HEREDITARY   NATIVE
INBORN   BUILT-IN   EASY

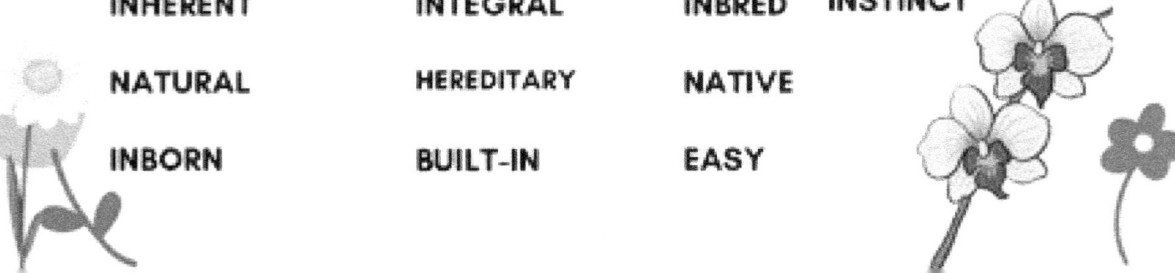

ORCHID

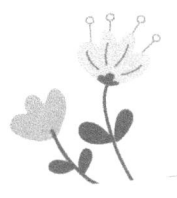

DAY TEN
SELF-LOVE

"Accepting yourself fully, treating yourself with kindness and respect, and nurturing your growth and wellbeing."

REFLECTION: Count your physical scars. Touch them and reflect on the fact that you survived it. Whatever tried to hurt you, you are still here and you intend to keep progressing. Count your biggest mistakes and errors. Now reflect on the lessons you learned from each mistake. Promise yourself that you will make better choices for your life.

 Self-Care Tip
Using the journal page for today describes what the best version of yourself looks like. Be specific and detailed because if you can see it, you can create it.

JOURNAL

_____
_____
_____
_____
_____
_____
_____

Love Day10

Can you find the words hidden in the puzzle?

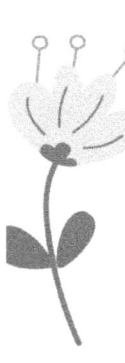

A	F	F	E	C	T	I	O	N	C	I	A
R	D	E	V	O	T	I	O	N	O	N	P
D	I	O	O	P	P	S	H	C	E	T	P
O	G	U	R	V	I	H	Y	I	O	I	R
U	N	N	A	A	N	O	I	N	G	M	E
R	I	S	L	M	T	L	I	V	E	A	C
E	O	Y	C	A	M	I	T	Y	I	C	I
A	N	S	Q	T	M	E	O	E	T	Y	A
M	W	E	I	Y	A	T	P	N	E	U	T
O	F	O	N	D	N	E	S	S	C	E	I
R	I	S	H	A	Y	E	A	N	K	A	O
A	T	T	A	C	H	M	E	N	T	Y	N

AFFECTION	**ATTACHMENT**	**FONDNESS**	**ARDOUR**
ADORATION	**INTIMACY**	**AMITY**	
DEVOTION	**APPRECIATION**	**AMOR**	

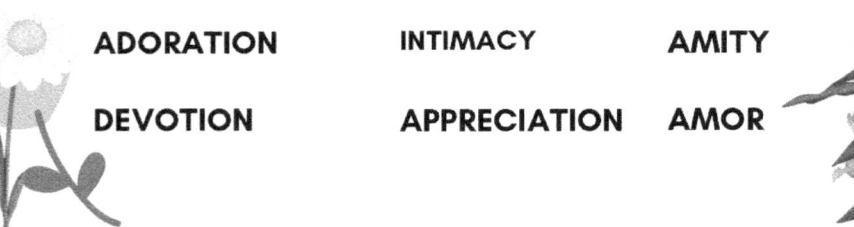

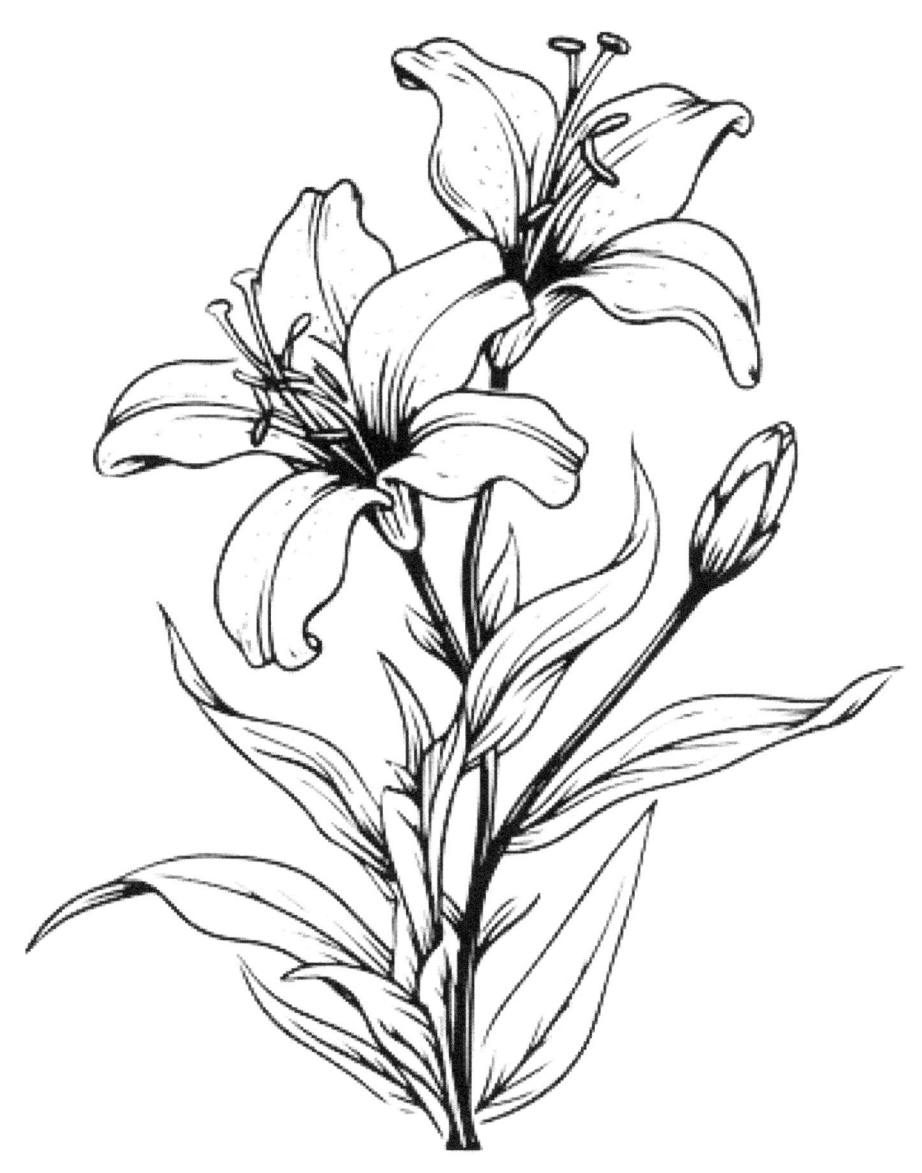

STARGAZER LILLY

DAY ELEVEN
YOU CAN BREAK THE CURSE

As a curse-breaker, The Most High has gifted you the power to take back anything the enemy ever stole from you and your family. You can break negative behaviors, attitudes and word curses. You are the Restorer! The Bible says in Luke 10:19 "Behold, I give unto you power to tread on serpents and scorpions, and over all the power of the enemy: and nothing shall by any means hurt you.

REFLECTION: What needs to be restored in your life or in your family?

 Self-Care Tip
This is a challenge. Turn off your phone, radio, television, all electronics and sit still for 15 – 30 minutes. Stay awake, allow yourself to relax and be open to receive what the quiet and stillness brings to your mind.

JOURNAL

_____
_____
_____
_____
_____
_____
_____

Restorer Day 11

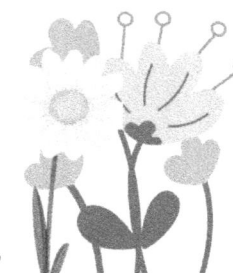

Can you find the words hidden in the puzzle?

```
R E H A B I L I T A T E
E E M C B E A R D O W N
C I B O P U S H C E N I
O G U U P G R A D E N C
N R N A I E O I N G I S
S E S L M L L I V E K N
T N S I R M D L U S O D
R E P A I R E C O V E R
U W E I M H T P K E U R
C C O V E R H A U L E D
T I R E V A M P N K A E
M E N D V E L R I T Y R
```

RECONSTRUCT	REHABILITATE	REBUILD	UPGRADE
REPAIR	OVERHAUL	RECOVER	
MEND	RENEW	REVAMP	

TULIP

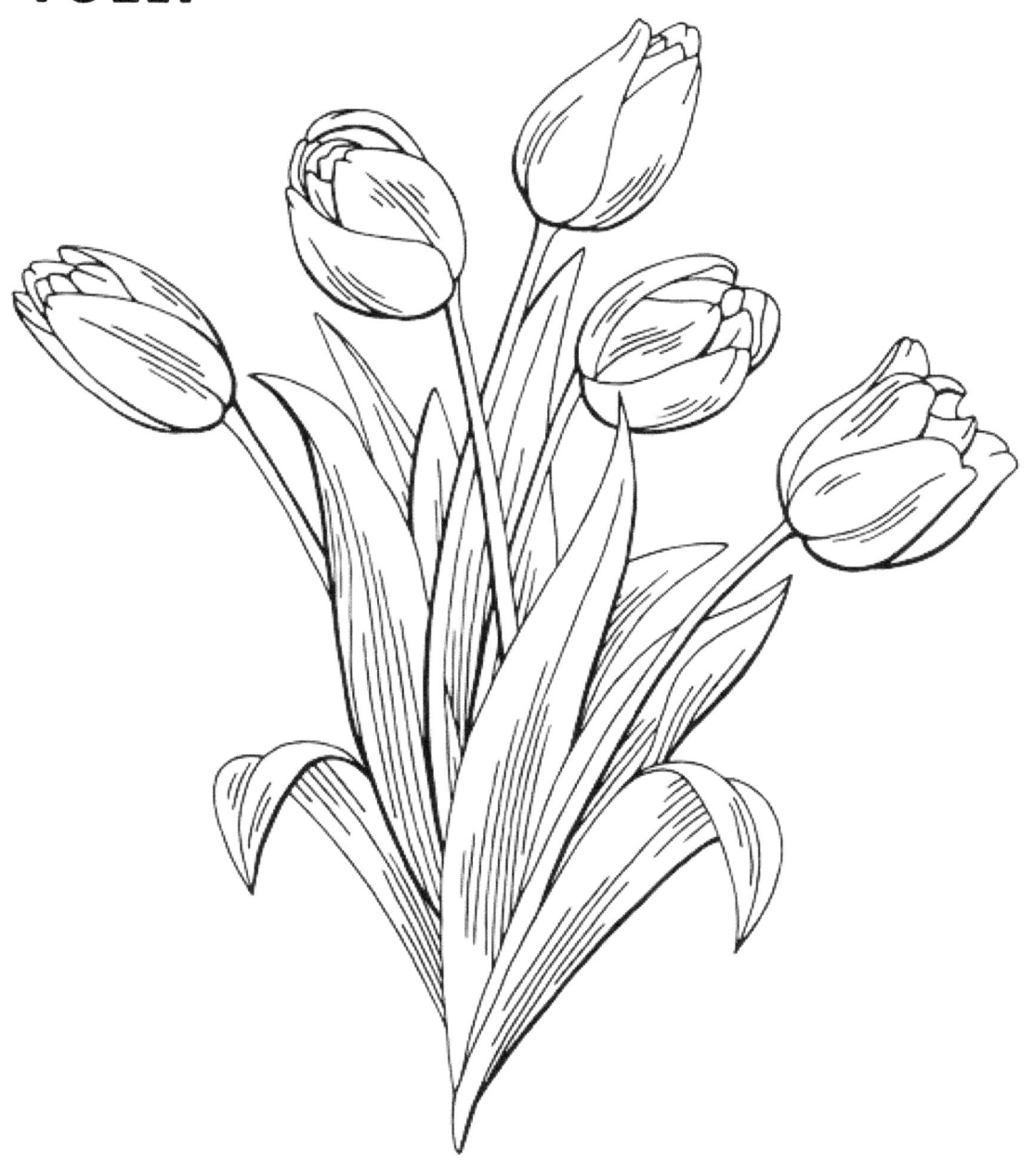

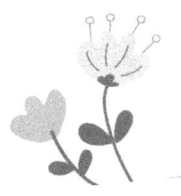

DAY TWELVE
JOURNEY

"An act of traveling from one place to another."

REFLECTION: There are times in our lives when we have to travel backwards in order to go forward. Although it may be painful, there's beauty waiting in exchange for those ashes. Take a journey back to your inner child to clarify some things, resolve the unresolved and apologize if needed.

Self-Care Tip
Using the journal page, write down your favorite scripture or quote. Have a conversation with yourself and discuss how these words impact you. Take a moment to review your life's journey. What have you overcome? What have you survived?

JOURNAL

_____

_____

_____

_____

_____

_____

_____

_____

Journey Day 12

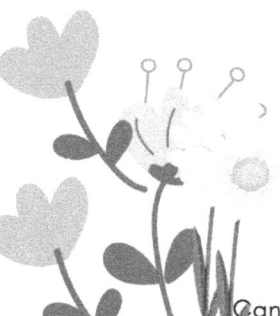
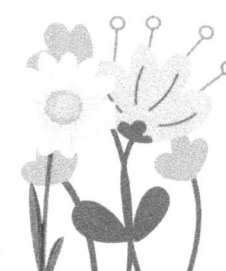

Can you find the words hidden in the puzzle?

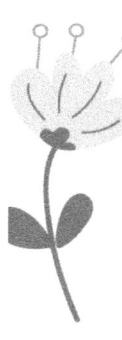

```
E X P L O R A T I O N E
X E M C A M P A I G N N
P I L G R I M A G E N I
E X O D U S Q U E S T C
D R N A I D O I N G I S
I E S L M V L I V E K N
T N S I R V O Y A G E D
I E P A D V E N T U R E
O W E I M T T P K E U R
N C O V E U H A U L E D
T R I P V R M P N K A E
M G N I L E V A R T Y R
```

EXPEDITION   PILGRIMAGE   ADVENTURE   CAMPAIGN

TRIP   QUEST   EXODUS

VOYAGE   TRAVELING   EXPLORATION

DAHLIA

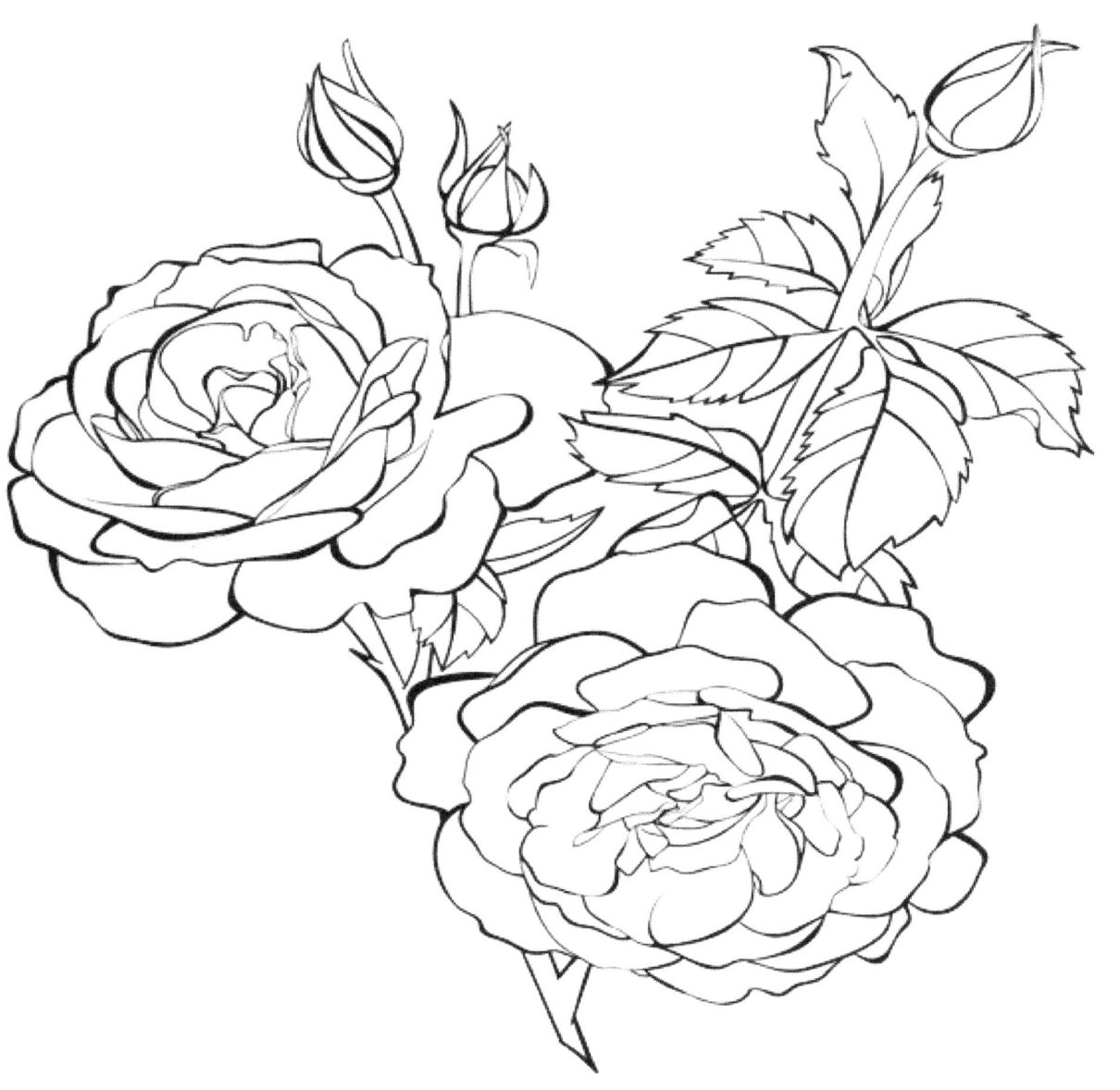

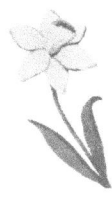

DAY THIRTEEN
OVERCOMER

"A person who overcomes something: one who succeeds in dealing with or gaining control of some problem or difficulty."

REFLECTION: Face your fears. What is your current struggle? How long have you been wrestling with this issue? Are you ready to quit? The good news is as of right now, you have overcome every struggle that tried to stop you. You're a winner, even if you didn't know it.

 Self-Care Tip
Let your imagination run wild. If you could travel to any place in the world, where would you go and why?

JOURNAL

_____
_____
_____
_____
_____
_____
_____
_____
_____

Courage
Day 13

Can you find the words hidden in the puzzle?

```
A S S U R A N C E A T F
P E M C B V A L O R W O
L I B O P U S H C E N R
O G U U P G R A D E N T
M R N A I E O I N G G I
B R A V E R Y I V E A T
T V I R T U E L U S L U
R A P A I R M R O L A D
U L E I M H E P K E N E
C O N V I C T I O N T D
T F E A R L E S S K R E
M E N D V E L R I T Y R
```

BRAVERY   CONVICTION   VIRTUE   FEARLESS

APLOMB   FORTITUDE   GALANTRY

ASSURANCE VALOR   METEL

DAFFODIL

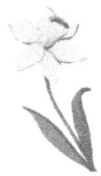

DAY FOURTEEN
MOVE OUT OF YOUR OWN WAY

"There's nothing stopping you but you. Whatever you believe about yourself, will come true. So, if you say "I can, I will, I have the victory." Those are the experiences that you will manifest. On the other hand, if you are habitually saying "I can't, I am not enough, I've never been able to." That is the future that you are creating for yourself."

REFLECTION: Get out of your own way. Recommended reading. "The Mountain is You" by Brianna Wiest.

 Self-Care Tip
Do you know how special you are? Do you know that The Most High considers you HIS treasured possession? Write down ten things about you that are special.

Deuteronomy 14:2, for you are a people holy to the Lord your God. Out of all the peoples on the face of the earth, the Lord has chosen you to be his treasured possession. Rephrase this scripture in your own words. Repeat it to yourself until it feels real.

JOURNAL

_____

_____

_____

_____

_____

_____

Move
Day 14

Can you find the words hidden in the puzzle?

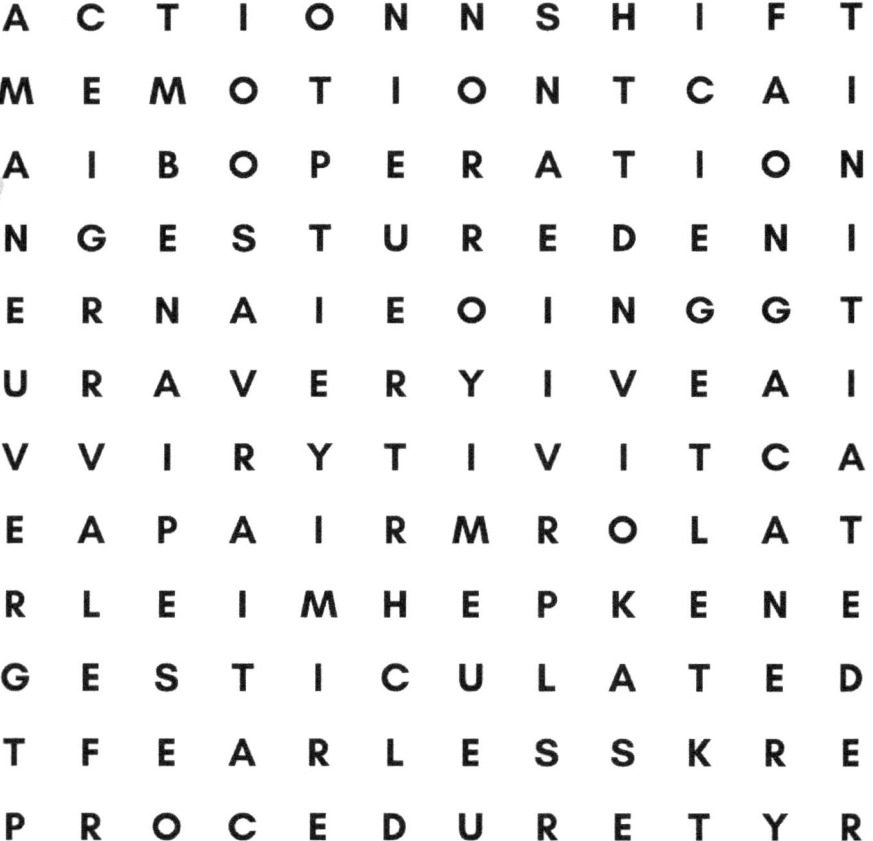

ACTION	ACTIVITY	SHIFT	INITIATE
MANEUVER	MOTION	GESTICULATE	
GESTURE	OPERATION	PROCEDURE	

PERIWINKLE

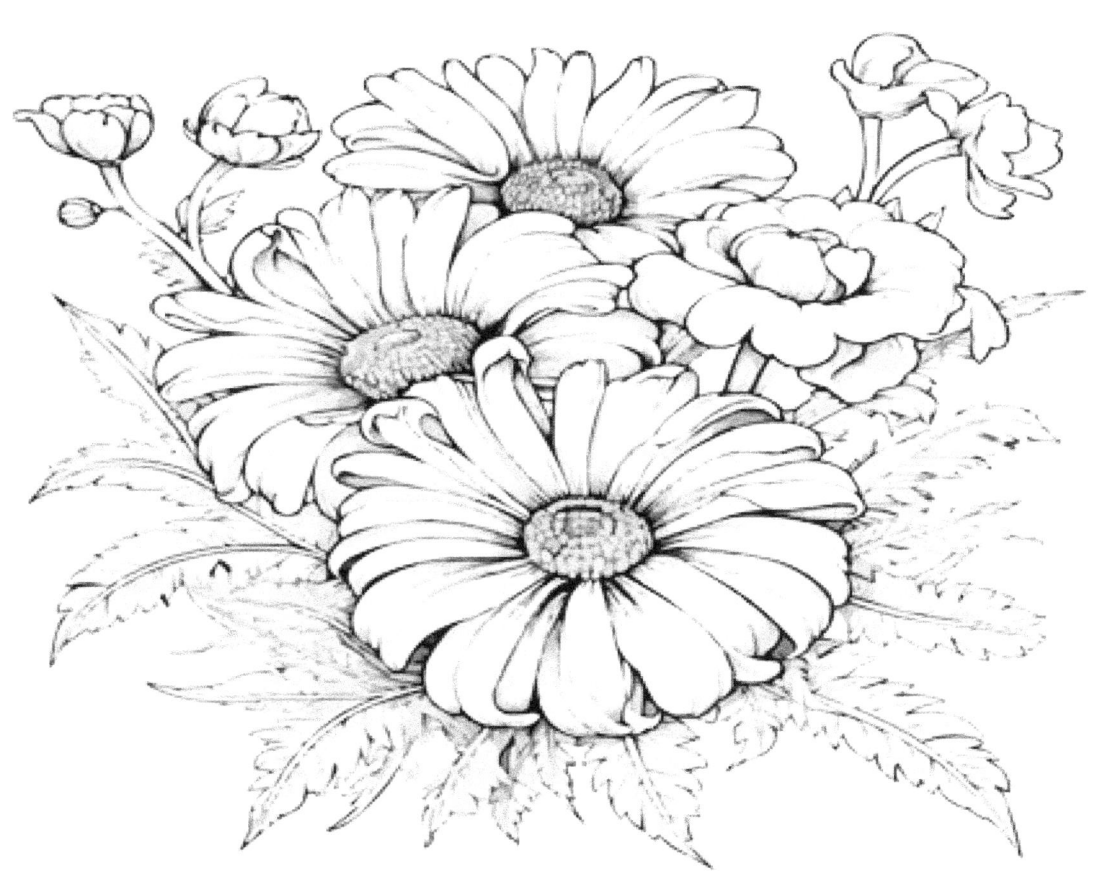

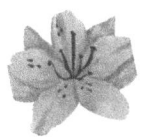

DAY FIFTEEN
VICTORY

"An act of defeating an enemy or opponent in a battle, game, or other competition."

REFLECTION: Celebrate yourself for whatever you have accomplished today. It doesn't matter what other people think. You know how hard it was and yet you won the battle. Victory is yours.

 Self-Care Tip
Today is grounding day. Find a patch of grass, dirt or sand. Remove your shoes and place your feet on the ground. Taking deep breaths, squeeze your toes back and forth and allow the earth to pull any negative energy or activity from your body. If you choose, write down the feeling afterwards.

JOURNAL

_____
_____
_____
_____
_____
_____
_____
_____

Victory Day 15

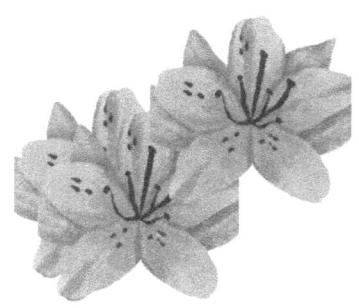

Can you find the words hidden in the puzzle?

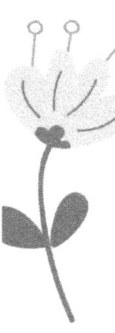

```
C O N Q U E S T E A T A
P R I Z E V W I N T W C
L I B O P U S H C T N C
O G U U P G R A D A N O
M R N A I E O I N I G M
G L O R Y R Y I V N A P
T R I U M P H F E A T L
R A P A I R M R O L A I
U L E I M S S E C C U S
C O N V I C T I O N T H
T F E A R L E S S K R E
M E E V E I H C A T Y R
```

TRIUMPH	**SUCCESS**	**CONQUEST**	**PRIZE**
ACCOMPLISH	**ATTAIN**	**WIN**	
ACHIEVE	**FEAT**	**GLORY**	

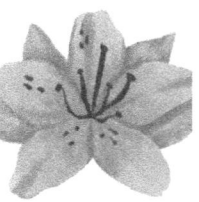

AZALEA

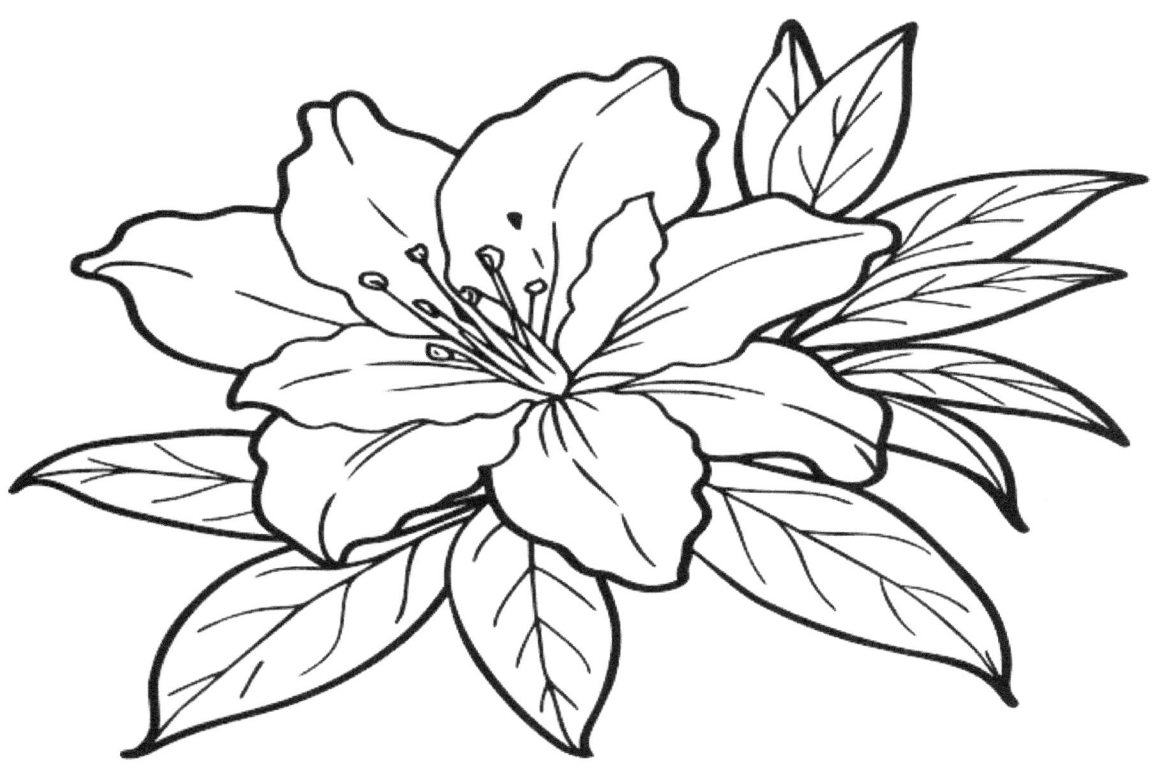

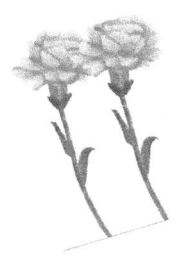

DAY SIXTEEN
What's for you will find you.

"What you seek is seeking you." ~ *Rumi*

REFLECTION: What's for you will be yours. The Universe will make sure you get your due. What have you been waiting for?

 Self-Care Tip
Take a walk today. If you're outside, be intentional about inhaling and exhaling the fresh air.

JOURNAL

_____
_____
_____
_____
_____
_____
_____
_____
_____
_____

Found Day 16

 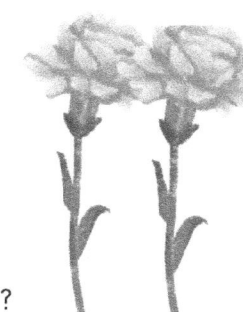

Can you find the words hidden in the puzzle?

```
I D E V E L O P F O R M
N L A U N C H I N R W O
S I B O P U S H C E N R
T G U U P G R A D E N T
I R N A E T A I T I N I
T R A B E G I N V E A T
U V I R T U E L U S L U
T A P A I R M R O L A D
E S T A R T C R E A T E
C O N V I C T I O N T D
T F E O R I G I N A T E
M E S T A B L I S H Y R
```

ESTABLISH   FORM   ORIGINATE   DEVELOP

LAUNCH   START   INSTITUTE

BEGIN   INITIATE   CREATE

CARNATION

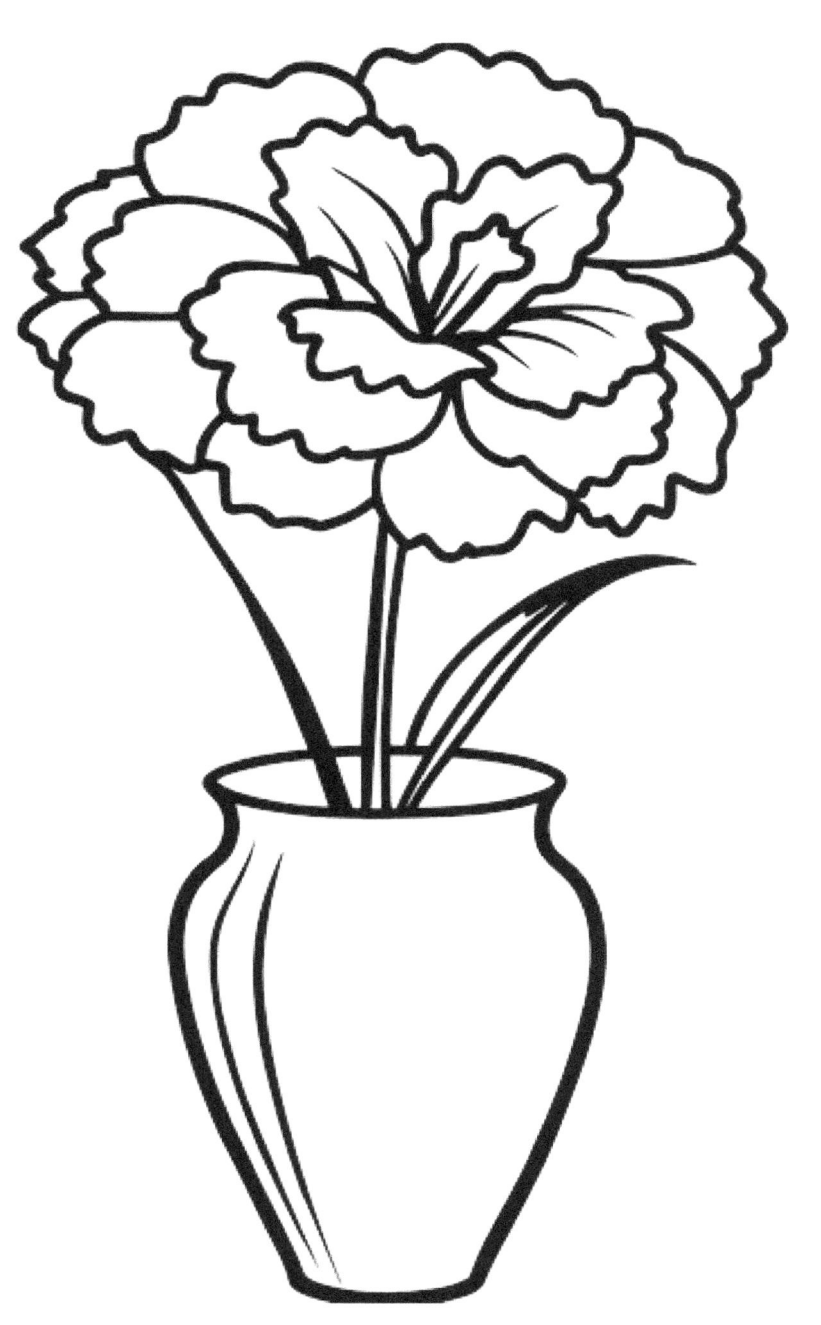

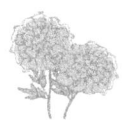

DAY SEVENTEEN
KEEP YOUR INNER GARDEN HEALTHY

"A healthy, fruitful garden requires some tools, hard work and fertilizer. A healthy abundant life will also require the right tools and effort. It will take digging into the soil of your heart and getting dirty every now and then."

REFLECTION: Think of what it takes to have a healthy garden. Good soil, water, sun, pruning and even your fertilizer, which is your mess. What is currently representing these tools in your life garden?

 Self-Care Tip
This is a challenge. Be intentional about clearing a space in your home, car, job, closet, kitchen drawer etcetera. Clearing physical space makes room to receive spiritually and mentally. Once you're done, write down how the space looks, feels and smells to you. Enjoy!

JOURNAL

_____

_____

_____

_____

_____

_____

_____

Healthy Day 17

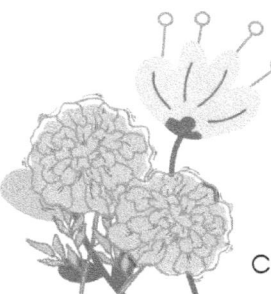

Can you find the words hidden in the puzzle?

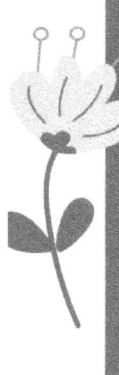

F	I	T	U	S	U	O	R	O	G	I	V
H	E	A	R	T	Y	A	W	E	L	L	O
L	I	B	O	R	U	S	H	C	E	N	R
O	G	U	U	O	G	R	A	D	E	N	T
F	I	N	E	N	E	O	I	N	G	T	B
B	R	A	V	G	R	Y	I	V	E	H	L
T	V	I	R	T	U	E	L	U	S	R	O
R	A	P	A	C	T	I	V	E	L	I	O
U	L	E	I	M	H	E	P	K	E	V	M
C	O	N	V	I	C	T	I	O	N	I	I
T	F	E	A	R	L	E	S	S	K	N	N
F	L	O	U	R	I	S	H	I	N	G	G

WELL **FINE** **FIT** **FLOURISHING**

HEARTY **THRIVING** **BLOOMING**

STRONG **VIGOROUS** **ACTIVE**

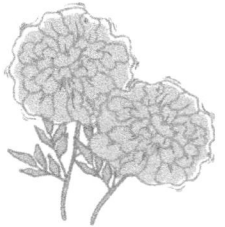

MARIGOLD

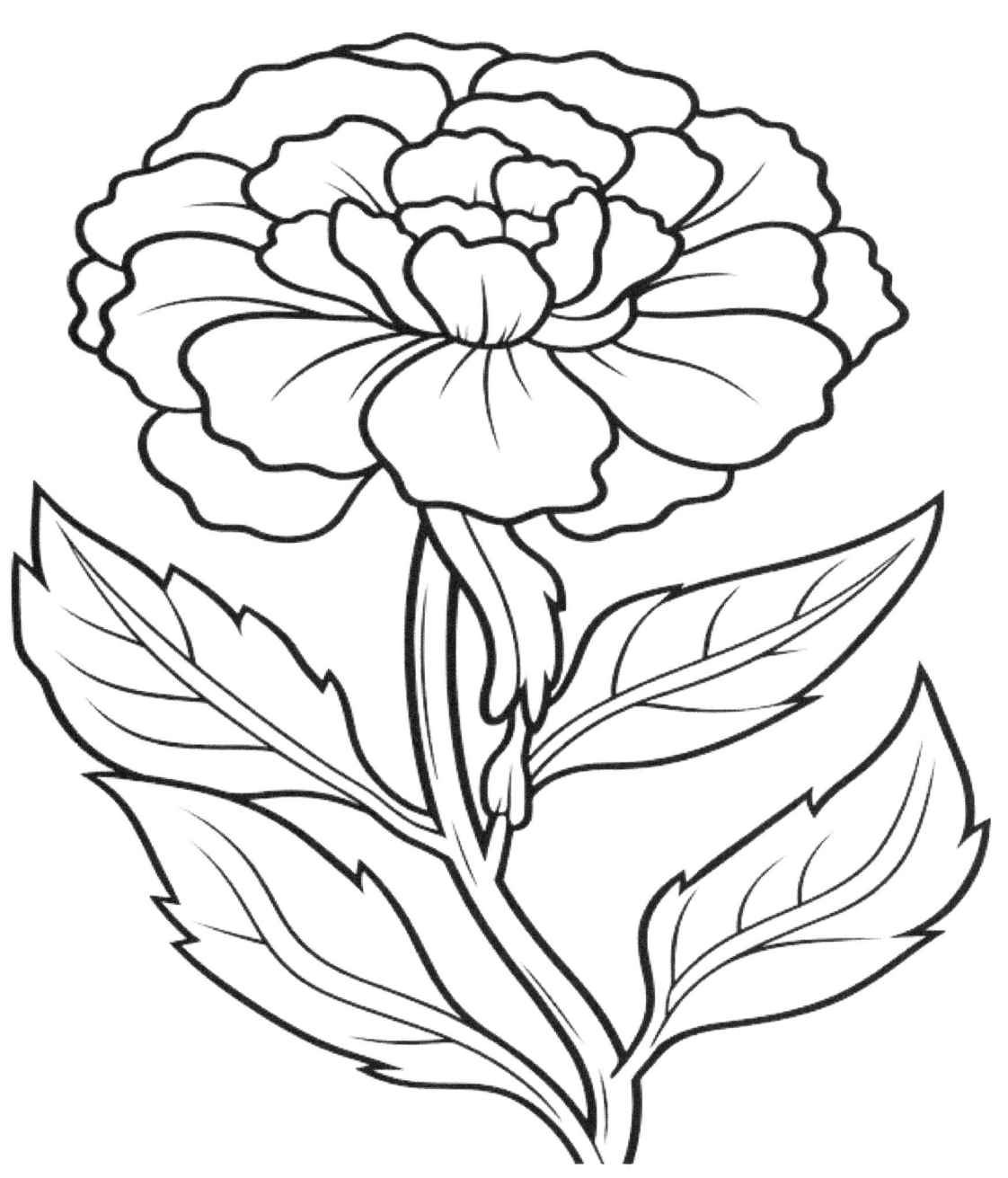

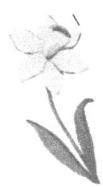

DAY EIGHTEEN
YOUR CELLS HAVE MEMORY

"Speaking to your cells in a positive manner on a daily basis changes the course of your thoughts and life. Be careful of the words you speak over yourself. Your soul is always listening to what you say and doesn't know if you're joking when you speak negatively. Everything you say about yourself will become a reality."

REFLECTION: Would it hurt you to start speaking positively about yourself and your life? Give it a try and see the results for yourself? Where do you want to start first?

Self-Care Tip
Make your own body scrub.

RECIPE
One cup sea salt

One cup sugar

1/2 a cup Organic oil such as Olive oil, Almond oil, Rose oil

A few drops of essential oil such as Lemon, Rose, Lavender.
Mix the ingredients together in a bowl.

Once the consistency is what you like, hop in the shower and apply the scrub to soften any rough areas on your body.

Use your fingers or a washcloth, scooping out a quarter size of the scrub and use slow circular motions to exfoliate the area, then rinse the scrub off.

This recipe may be too rough for your face but it is perfect for the neck, elbows, hands, knees and feet. Note the difference you feel in your skin after the treatment.

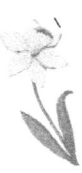

JOURNAL: _____

Memory Day 18

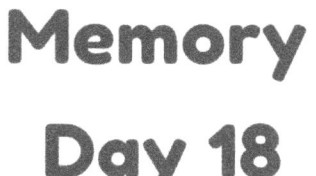

Can you find the words hidden in the puzzle?

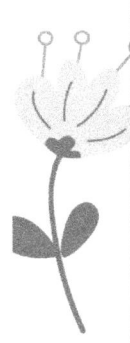

```
A R S K C A B H S A L F
N E M A I G L A T S O N
A M B O P U S H C E N T
M I N D S E Y E D E N C
N N N A I E O I N G G E
E I A V E R Y I V E A P
S S I R E C A L L S L S
I C N O I T N E T E R O
S E R E M E M B E R N R
C O N V I C T I O N T T
T R E M I N I S C E R E
H I N D S I G H T T Y R
```

REMEMBER   **RETENTION**   **MINDSEYE**   **RECALL**

REMINISCE   **FLASHBACK**   **NOSTALGIA**

RETROSPECT   **HINDSIGHT**   **ANAMNESIS**

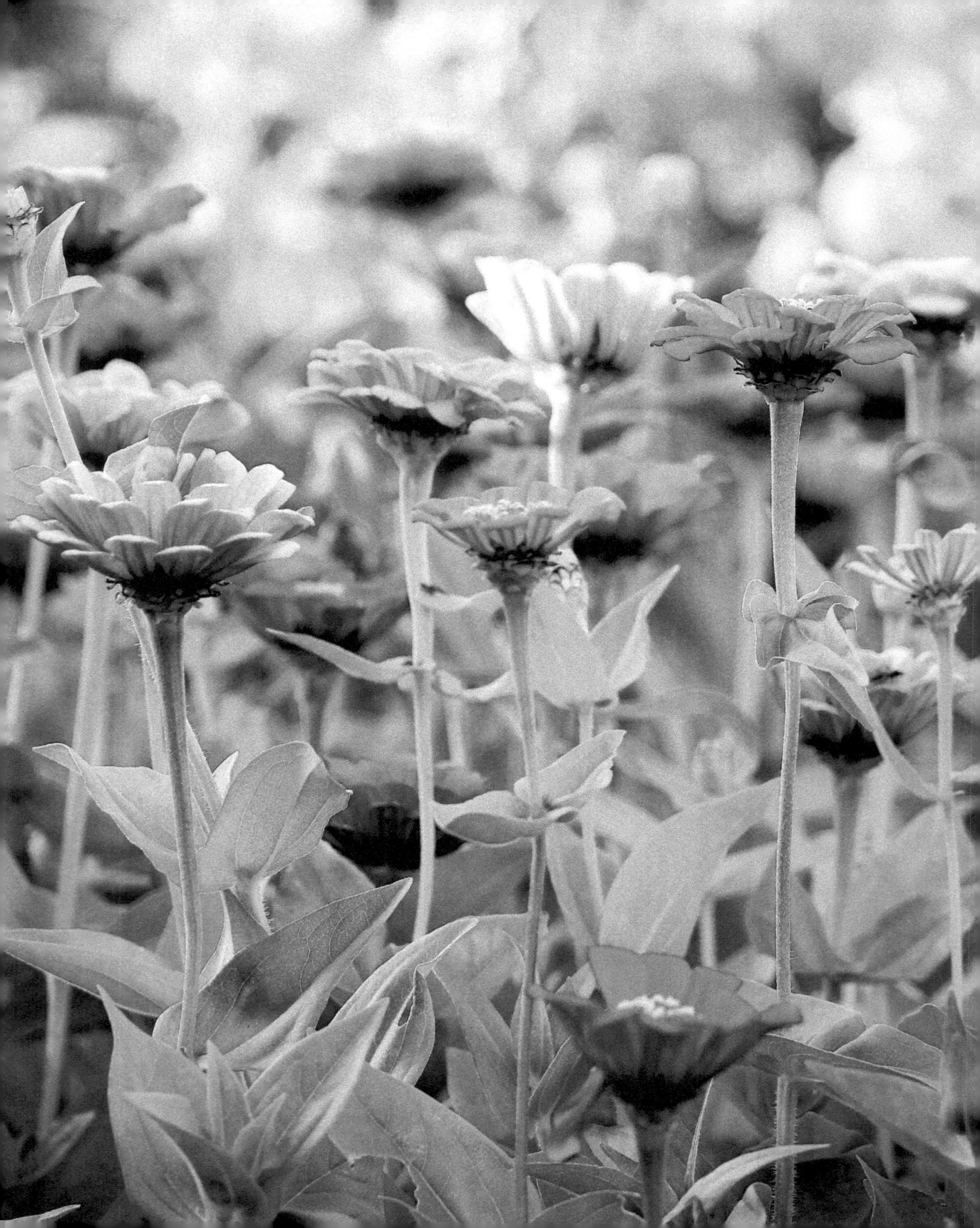

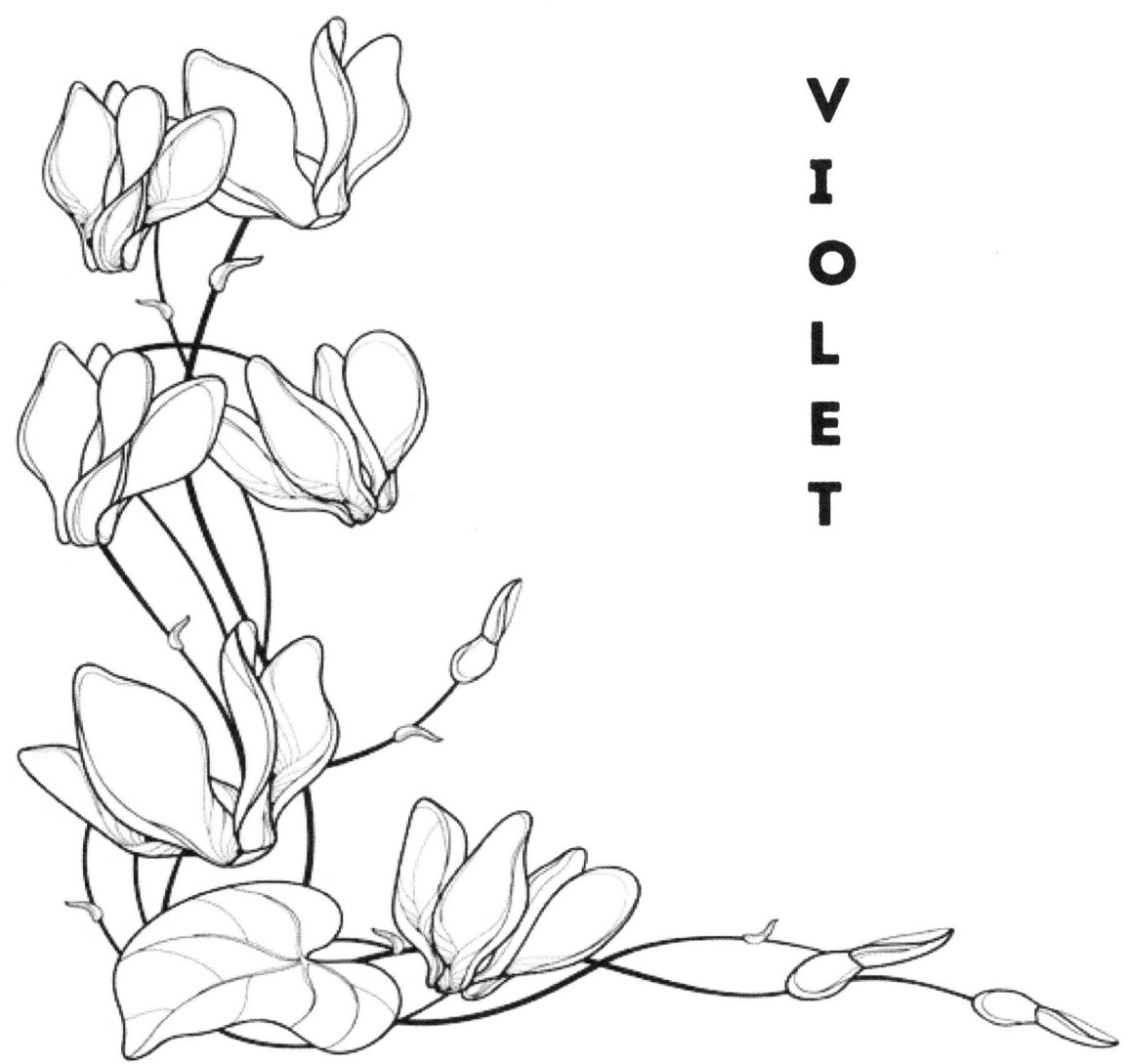

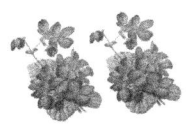

DAY NINETEEN
SPEAK GOOD TO YOURSELF

""Speaking to your cells daily changes the course of your thoughts and life. Be careful of the words you speak over yourself. Your soul is always listening to you. Your soul doesn't know if you're joking when you speak negatively about yourself. Everything that you say about yourself will be made true."

REFLECTION: Encourage yourself, the same way you encourage others. Through your words, you can affirm, validate and encourage yourself. The words you speak to yourself are sacred; make every word count.

 Self-Care Tip
It's Entrepreneur Day. Pray for your own business, and pray for the business of others. Today make an effort to try and patronize a business that is run by an entrepreneur who you personally know.

JOURNAL

_____
_____
_____
_____
_____
_____

Words Day 19

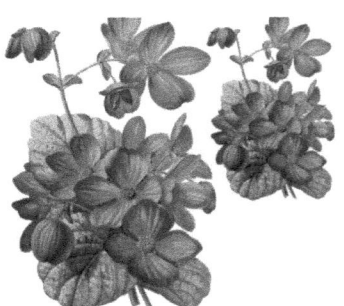

Can you find the words hidden in the puzzle?

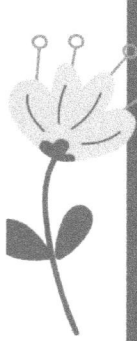

A	S	E	U	G	O	L	A	I	D	T	F
C	O	N	V	E	R	S	E	T	I	W	E
H	I	B	O	P	U	S	H	C	S	N	T
A	G	U	U	P	G	R	A	D	C	D	A
T	R	N	A	I	E	O	I	N	U	I	L
B	R	A	V	E	R	Y	I	V	S	S	U
T	V	I	R	T	U	E	L	U	S	C	B
A	A	P	A	R	L	E	Y	O	I	O	A
L	L	E	I	M	H	E	P	K	O	U	F
K	O	N	V	I	C	T	I	O	N	R	N
T	D	E	B	A	T	E	S	S	K	S	O
C	O	M	M	U	N	I	C	A	T	E	C

COMMUNICATE

CONVERSE   **DISCOURSE**   **TALK**

DIALOGUE   **DISCUSSION**   **DEBATE**

CHAT   **CONFABULATE**   **PARLEY**

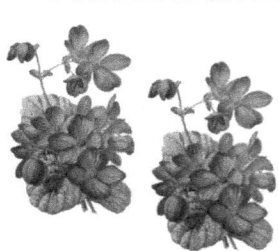

BEGONIA

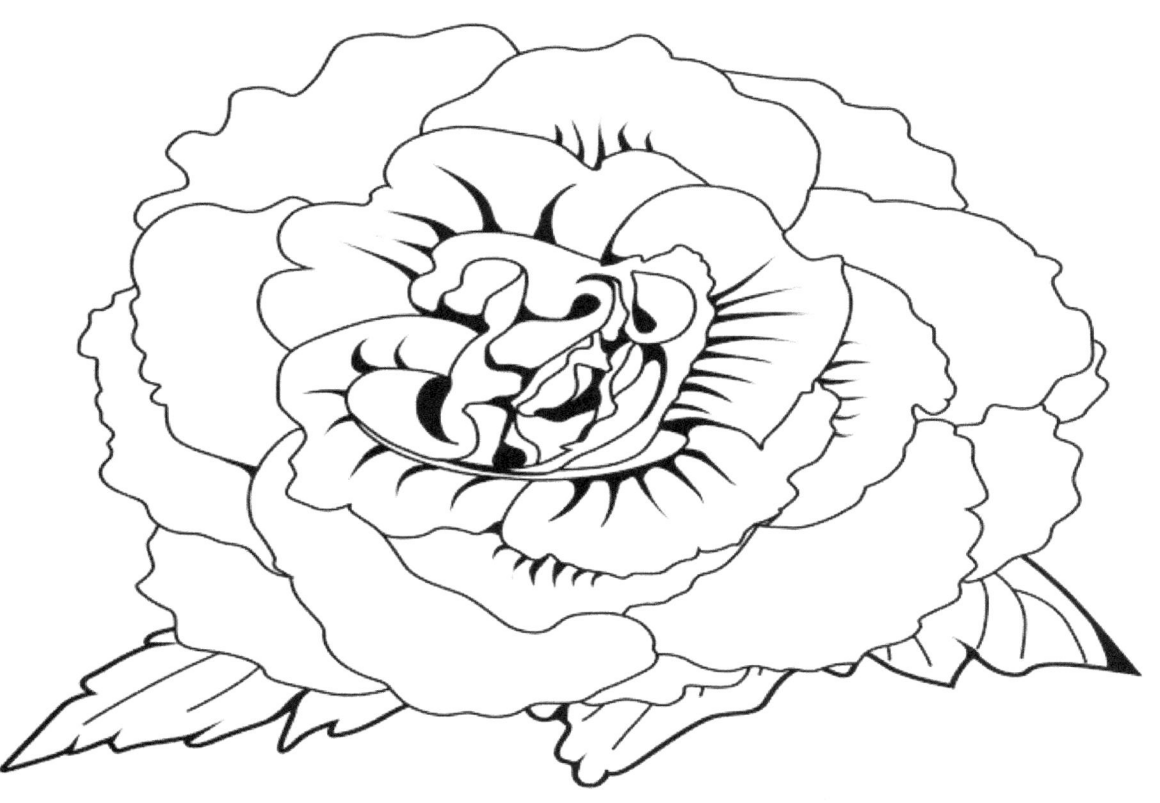

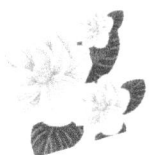

DAY TWENTY
PURPOSE

"The reason for which something is done or created or for which something exists:"

REFLECTION: Live Your Purpose.
The two most important days of your life are the day you were born and the day you find out why. – Mark Twain

Have you discovered your life's purpose yet?

Do you have any ideas about what you should be doing?

If not, it's okay, because there's great news. You can be intentional with your words and actions; every single day – on purpose.

 Self-Care Tip
Let's practice fasting today. Choose your fasting window, what you will be fasting from? What words and/or prayers will you be speaking into your life during your fast to be effective and receive revelations?

JOURNAL

_____

_____

_____

_____

_____

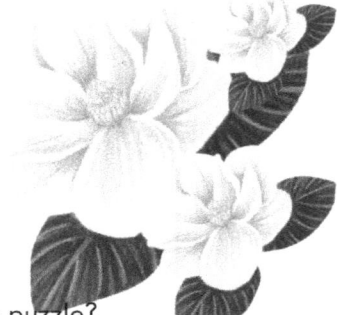

Purpose
Day 20

Can you find the words hidden in the puzzle?

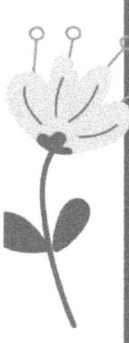

```
O B J E C T I V E A T D
P E M C B V A L O R W I
L I B A P U S H C E N R
O G U U P G R A D E N E
M R N S I E O I N G G C
B R A E E R Y P O I N T
T V I R T U E L U S L I
R A P A I R M A O L A O
M L E I N T E N T E N N
I D E A I C T I O N T D
A F E A R L E S S K R E
M L A O G S D N U O R G
```

GOAL	IDEA	POINT	GROUNDS
AIM	INTENT	CAUSE	
OBJECTIVE	PLAN	DIRECTION	

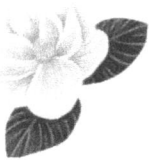

M
A
G
N
O
L
I
A

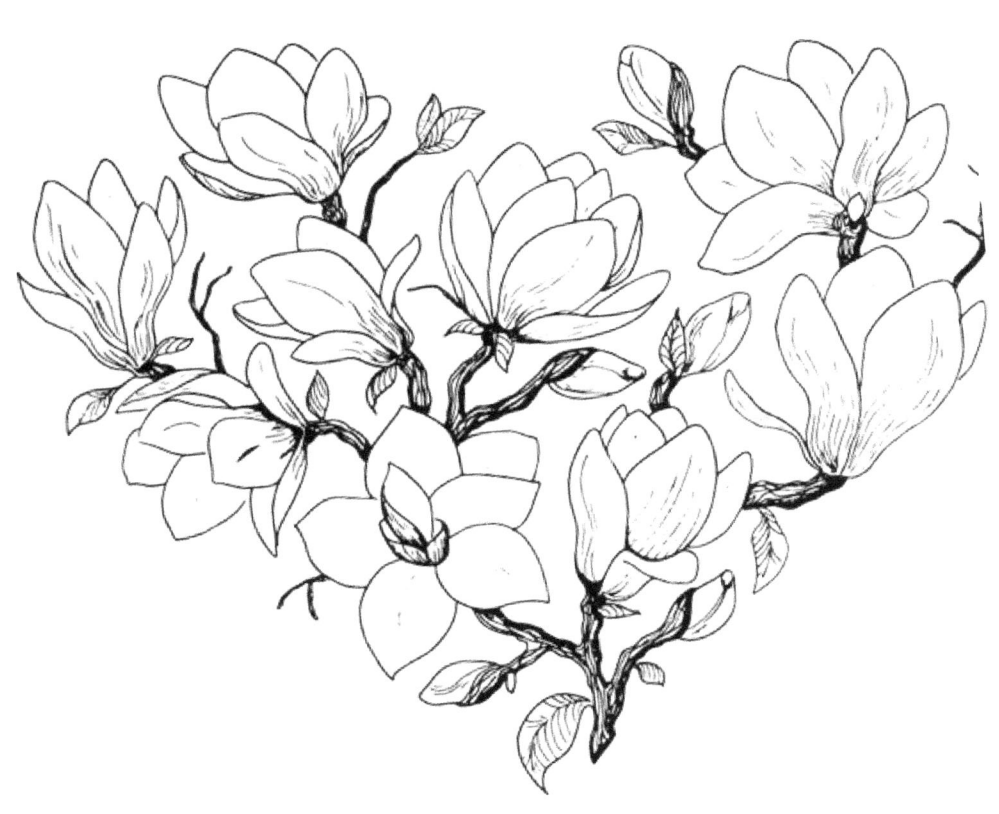

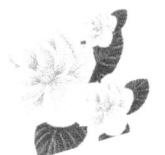

DAY TWENTY-ONE

BET ON YOURSELF AND I BET YOU WILL WIN

Have you ever consciously affirmed yourself; either out loud or silently? Try saying "I choose me", "I am worthy", "I am enough", "I can do anything I put my mind to."

REFLECTION: If you could challenge yourself to do anything, what would it be? Betting on you is an intentional decision to make a commitment to yourself and follow through until the task is completed.

 Self-Care Tip
Intentionally try a vegan dish today. Using the journal page, write about the taste, texture, smell. Did you like it? Would you try it again? How was the overall experience?

JOURNAL

_____

_____

_____

_____

_____

_____

_____

_____

Winning Day 21

Can you find the words hidden in the puzzle?

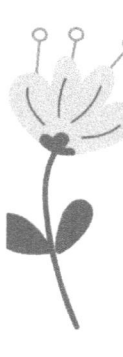

```
A S S U R A N C E A T F
P U M C B V A L O R W O
G C B O P U S H C E N R
N C H A M P I O N E N T
I E N A I E O I N G G I
R S Y R O T C I V E A T
E S I T R I U M P H L U
U F I R S T M B O L A D
Q L E I M H E P K E N E
N O U N B E A T E N T D
O B E S T L E S S K R E
C P O T V L E A D I N G
```

VICTORY	SUCCESS	UNBEATEN	LEADING
TRIUMPH	CONQUERING	BEST	
CHAMPION	FIRST	TOP	

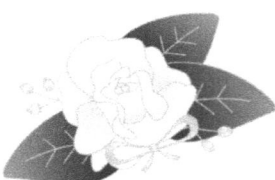

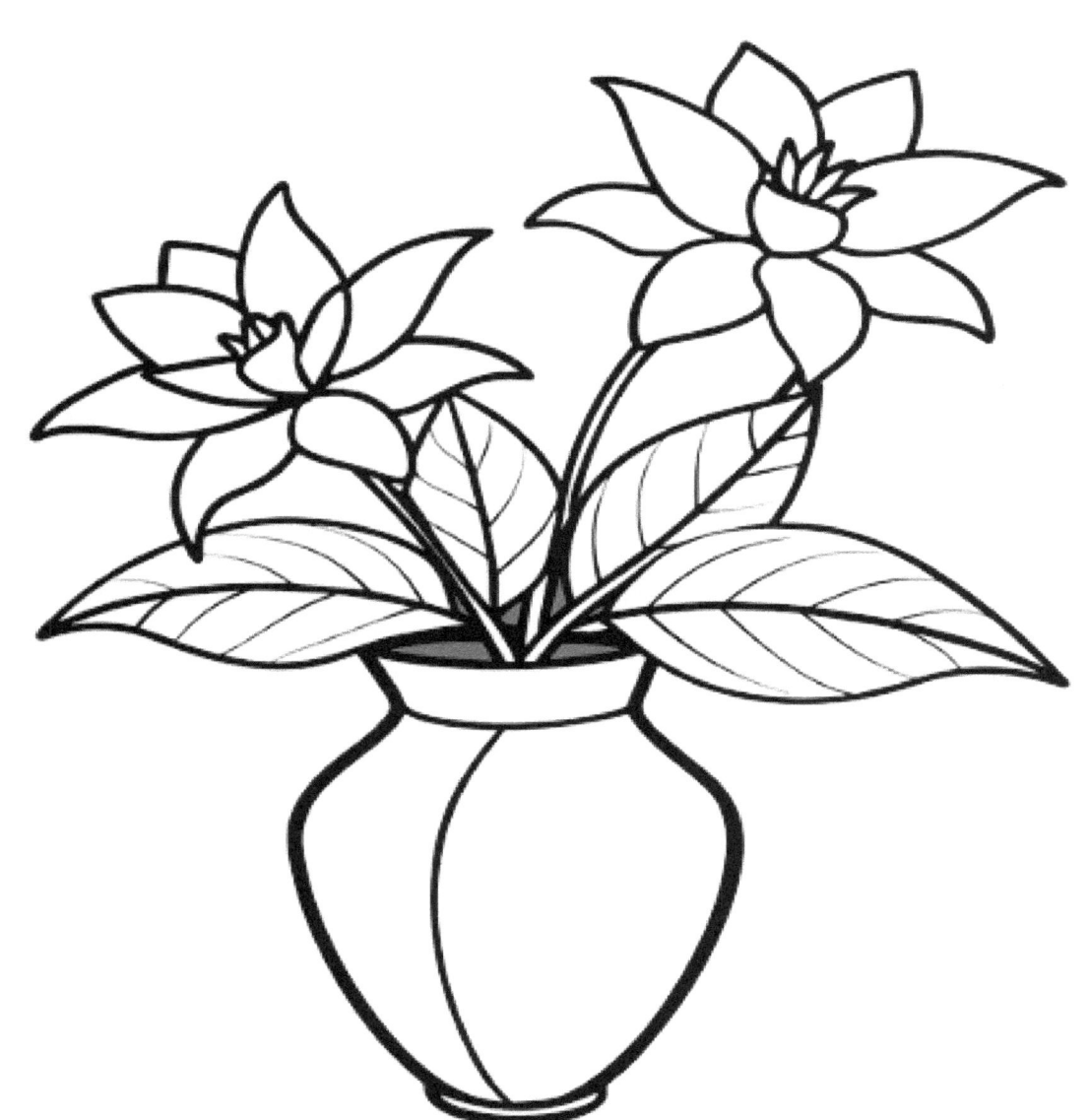

ACKNOWLEDGMENT

I WANT TO FIRST AND FOREMOST ACKNOWLEDGE THE MOST HIGH – ELOHIM, THE CREATOR. IT IS HE WHO GAVE ME THIS CONCEPT WHILE WALKING THROUGH THE STORE ONE AFTERNOON. I LOOKED AT A WORD SEARCH PUZZLE (ONE OF MY FAVORITE PAST TIMES) AND SAID OUT LOUD– "I'VE NEVER SEEN A WORD SEARCH FOR SELF-CARE. HMM, OKAY, I'LL CREATE ONE." THIS ACTIVITY BOOK WAS CONCEIVED IN THAT MOMENT.

I HAVE TO SHOUT OUT MY FRIEND, JONATHAN "SHUG" BILLUPS. HE HAS CORRECTED, EDITED AND SUGGESTED THROUGHOUT THIS PROCESS. I APPRECIATE HIS HEART AND ENCOURAGEMENT TO ALWAYS WANT TO SEE ME WIN.

MONA WILLIAMS AND I HAD NO IDEA OF THE FUTURE RELATIONSHIP THAT YAHWEH HAD IN STORE FOR US WHEN WE MET YEARS AGO AT THE BLACK WOMEN'S EXPO. ONLY HE KNEW THE FUTURE PLANS FOR US TO COLLABORATE ON VARIOUS PROJECTS. THANK YOU, MONA, FOR YOUR BEAUTIFUL INTERIOR DESIGN OF THIS BOOK.

THANK YOU, JL WOODSON, OF WOODSON STUDIOS FOR ANOTHER BEAUTIFUL COVER.

WE ARE ALL BETTER, WHEN WORKING TOGETHER!
(PARAPHRASED FROM TONEAL JACKSON)

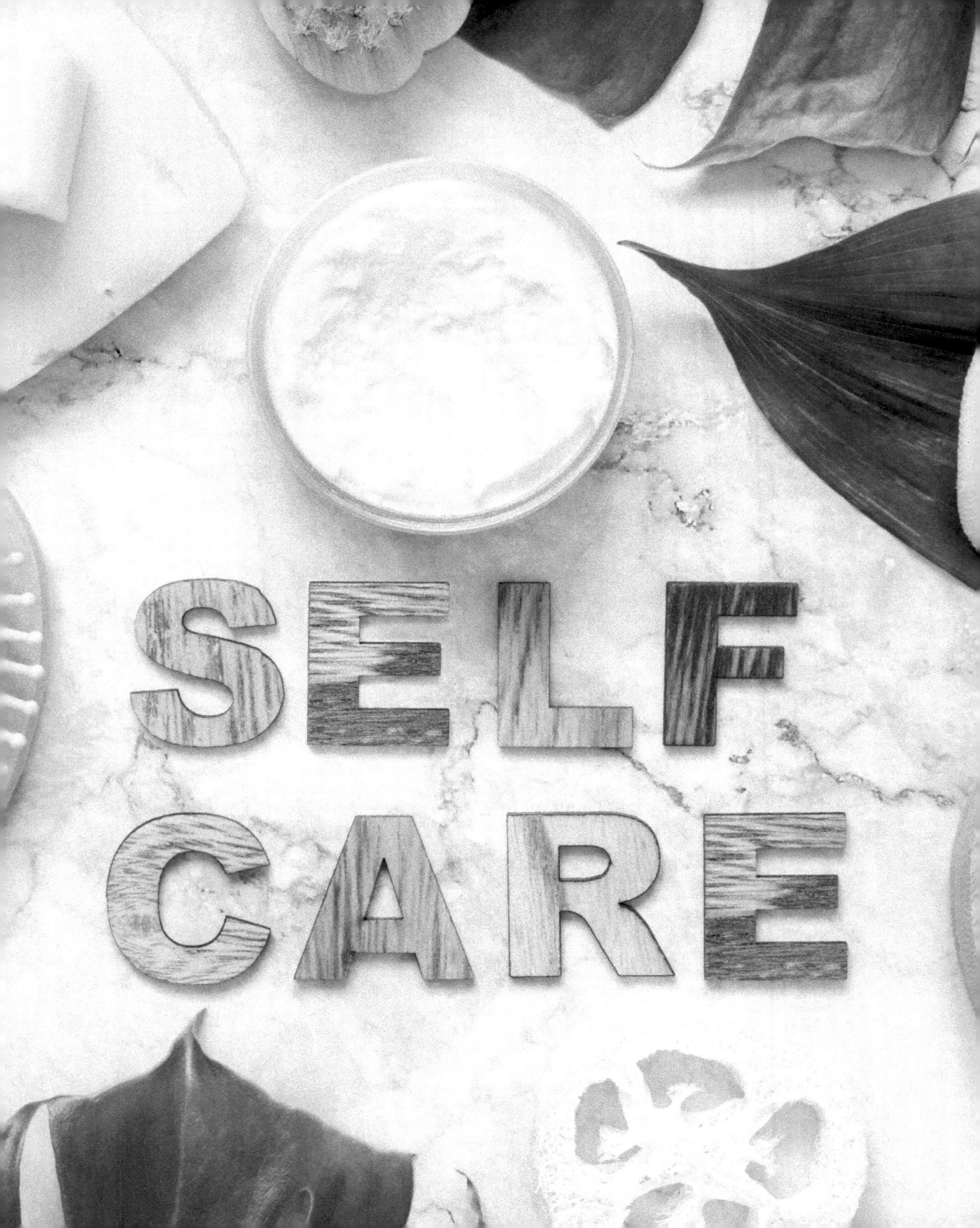

www.ingramcontent.com/pod-product-compliance
Lightning Source LLC
Chambersburg PA
CBHW042358070526
44585CB00029B/2989